Also by Sib

Fourteen D
The Fashion Police
My Perfect Wedding
Be Careful What You Wish For
How to Dump Your Boyfriend in the Men's Room (and
other short stories)
Trafficked: The Diary of a Sex Slave

About the author

Sibel Hodge is the author of bestselling romantic comedy
Fourteen Days Later. She has 8 cats and 1 husband. In her
spare time, she's Wonder Woman! When she's not out
saving the world from dastardly demons, she writes quirky
chick lit with a hefty dose of screwball comedy.

Her work has been shortlisted for the Harry Bowling Prize
2008, Highly Commended by the Yeovil Literary Prize
2009, Runner up in the Chapter One Promotions Novel
Comp 2009, and nominated Best Novel with Romantic
Elements in 2010 by The Romance Reviews. Her novella
Trafficked: The Diary of a Sex Slave has been listed as one
of the Top 40 Books About Human Rights by Accredited
Online Colleges.

For more information, please visit
http://www.sibelhodge.com/

The Baby Trap

Sibel Hodge

*This one's dedicated to my husband Brad,
for all your support and belief in me.*

Yesterday is history. Tomorrow is a mystery. And today? Today is a gift. That's why we call it the present." -- Babatunde Olatunji

Prologue

Why is it that you spend most of your young adult life trying not to get pregnant, and yet when you actually want to get pregnant, you can't? How annoying is that? Not to mention frustrating, depressing, soul-destroying, and numerous other feelings that I've experienced at one time or another in the last two years. I know I'm in danger of losing myself in a never-ending round of fertility treatment, wishing this time it's going to magically work. No, that's wrong. I've lost myself already. I've become a neurotic nutcase who's bored with life, boring, unsociable, and turning into a frump. What happened to the happy, carefree woman I used to be? The woman who used to enjoy life, have a laugh, appreciate her lot, and drink one too many bottles of wine at the weekends? Obsessed. Yes, that's what I am, but it's not my fault. It's this feeling that I can't explain. This desperate need inside me to have a baby. This urge that has completely turned my brain to single-train thoughts: Baby, baby, baby.

And as the years have gone on, I'm morphing into the ghost of myself. Someone who can't enjoy life because I'm too busy worrying and wondering when and if it's going to happen for me. I don't even recognize myself most of the time anymore. I'm constantly wishing for the end of my cycle to hurry up and arrive to see if I've hit the jackpot this time, and when it doesn't work, I'm constantly wishing for the middle of my cycle so I can ovulate and try again. I'm unable to feel whole and complete unless I have a son or daughter to hold.

So this year I have to take drastic action before I get sucked into a giant abyss of despair and can never get back.

I'm going to give it six more months of trying, and if I still can't get pregnant…well, that's it. I'm giving up. This is the last year I'm going through it. I've absolutely, definitely, positively made my mind up. I know I said that the last time, and the time before that, oh, and the time before that, but I really mean it this time.

Really.

Maybe really.

Nope. Really and truly, this year is going to be my year to give up trying for a baby.

I'm sick of people looking up my lady garden, prodding me, poking me. Doctors and nurses at the Assisted Conception Unit and friends looking at me with sympathy. I'm also sick of the following:

1) Having no spontaneous sex. It's not the same when you have to have precision-timed nookie. I'm also having to give precision-timed wanks to Karl in aid of sperm tests.

2) Leaving my legs hanging in the air after sex for ten minutes – although have been known to do it for up to forty as there are varying opinions on the length of time necessary.

3) Being obsessed about babies all the time.

4) Not having time for Karl and me anymore as always obsessing about babies. I'm worried we're drifting apart.

5) Being hormonal and moody from all the fertility drugs, and sometimes wanting to kill perfectly innocent people for no reason.

6) Bawling my eyes out every time I have my period (and countless other times, too).

7) Eating healthy organic food and giving up alcohol and smoking.

8) Constantly texting tarot card hotlines to find out if and when I will get pregnant (my mobile phone bill is the same as a small country's debt!).

9) Trying every alternative fertility treatment under the sun.

10) Isn't that enough reasons?

I always said I'd never write down my infertility journey, but I've changed my mind now. Actually, it was Poppy, whom I met online at the Fertility Friends website, who suggested it. We've got to know each other pretty well through emails and phone calls in the last two years. How can I describe Poppy? Hmm…if I'd met her in any normal circumstances she wouldn't have been my type of friend. She's a floaty, New Age, holistic type, who says she can see auras and talks about cosmic energy, Karma, and projecting positive thoughts to the Universe. Now, normally I'd burst into uncontrollable laughter if someone told me I had to imagine a bright white light of happiness radiating through my body to my ovaries, but I've done some pretty bizarre things in my quest to get pregnant, so maybe it's time I started listening to her and took her advice. What the hell, why not? What have I got to lose? I mean, the drugs and IVF don't seem to be working, so if I can finally have my little bundle of joy by chanting a few words and hugging a tree, why not give it a go? Although Karl will probably freak and think I've lost my mind completely after all the "ridiculous ideas" (as he calls them) I've come up with so far. I've gone from being someone totally unsuperstitious to someone who looks for signs everywhere. And I mean everywhere. Not to mention the fertility symbols and spells.

Anyway, Poppy told me that writing my story down is the first step to cosmic enlightenment (not entirely sure what that is, but it sounds nice). She explained that if I keep this journal, I'll be letting the Universe know exactly what I want and she (or he, not entirely what sex the Universe represents, although I think it's a she and will name her Zelda, which is a Universe-ish kind of name) will help me get rid of any negative energies surrounding me, unblock my chakras (whatever they are), and help me let go of my grief about being unable to get pregnant. OK, in a tiny little way it makes sense, but, of course, I can't tell that to Karl. He doesn't understand. And I can't help thinking that if all this

3

stuff she talks about could really work, then why isn't she pregnant yet, either?

But I'm game, and this is the last sliver of hope I can cling to. So on the first day of a brand new year, which Poppy said is the perfect time for cosmic alignment, you, my little pink diary with the silver clasp, will be my new friend. And if you can find time to poke the Universe and get her to grant my wish, then I'll be eternally grateful. Because if I can't get pregnant this time, I'll need to do something radical to fill this gaping hole in my life, and I'm scared of what that radical thing might be.

My Body Clock

It all started when I turned thirty-three. I woke up one Sunday morning and I could've sworn I heard a clock ticking. I prised open one sleepy eyelid, stuck together with caked mascara that I'd forgotten to take off again after another mad party. Maybe it was my head banging with a humongous hangover that was making the noise. I turned towards my husband Karl, snoring softly beside me with his mouth open, and groaned. Oops, big mistake! My head felt like someone was repeatedly hitting it with a sledgehammer. Probably not a good idea to actually move. Maybe I should just stay in bed all day. Yep, good idea.

Except the bloody ticking wouldn't shut up.

I knew it couldn't be the alarm clock on my bedside table because that had run out of batteries months ago. And it couldn't have been Karl's because he had a digital clock next to the bed. So what was it?

God, how much had I drunk last night? Was I hallucinating sounds? Whoa, I really needed to slow down on the wine next time.

I rolled out of bed, clutching my head in my hands, and wandered downstairs into the kitchen that overlooked the garden. Pouring a hefty glass of water to combat brain dehydration, I glugged it down in one go as I stared through hangover-induced blurry eyes at an oak tree outside.

What was that out there?

Instantly alert, my monster headache disappeared. I narrowed my eyes at a peculiar site in the garden. It was…what the hell was it? No, it couldn't be.

5

I unlocked the back door and tentatively crept towards the vision.

As I got closer, I couldn't believe my eyes.

It was a baby! Complete with a pink baby grow and a pink dummy, sucking on it with glee as it stared up at me with chubby cheeks and huge blue eyes.

What had I been drinking last night? Has someone spiked my drink at Amelia's party?

What kind of person could abandon a baby in someone's garden? This was unbelievable!

'You poor thing.' I reached out to pick it up and bring it inside the house and it disappeared.

Pfffft! Just like that. Vanished.

Karl found me two hours later, sitting at the farmhouse kitchen table, still in my fluffy pink pyjamas and giant slippers that looked like cows' faces, staring blankly at the garden.

'God, what a great night!' He kissed the top of my head and yawned. 'Want a coffee? I feel like I've swallowed a Brillo Pad.'

'Huh?' I said, not really hearing was he was saying.

'Coffee? Want one?' He rummaged around in the cupboards, pulling out mugs and a French press.

'Mmm.' I nodded absentmindedly.

He flicked the kettle on, lounged on the chair in front of me, and started chuckling. 'Do you remember dancing on the table last night? That was hilarious! You, Amelia, and Kerry doing a Coyote Ugly impression, flashing your knickers.'

I didn't answer. I was too busy worrying I had a brain tumour. That's what happened, wasn't it? I'd seen a programme about it once. People started hearing things and seeing things. Freaky things. Things that couldn't possibly be explained. Omigod, that was it. I was going to die! I was still young. I had my whole life ahead of me. Fun, mad shopping sprees, exotic holidays, lots of alcohol-induced partying (I'm not an alcoholic, honestly!). Except…I was getting this weird feeling. Suddenly all that stuff seemed

6

inconsequential – childish, even. I was thirty-three years old, and now I wanted…

'I want a baby!' I blurted out, not really knowing where the thought had come from. Maybe we'd been abducted by aliens on the way home last night and one of those sneaky guys had implanted a weird chip in my brain. It could happen. I watched *the X Files*, you know. Or was reaching thirty-three the new forty? Did you start having a midlife crisis, or, even worse, a nervous breakdown?

Karl's dark brown eyes sprang open and his jaw dropped. 'What?'

I adjusted myself in the chair, elbows on the table, leaning forward with an excited feeling simmering away beneath the surface. 'I want a baby.' A large grin had suddenly implanted itself on my face.

He ran a hand through his short dark hair. Now it was his turn to do the blank stare bit. 'Oh, right.' He rose from the table as if he hadn't heard me. 'Well, I need a coffee.' He poured the boiling water into the French press and brought it to the table with two mugs. As he flopped back down again, he said, 'Er…did I just hear you right?' He poked his fingers in his ears, as if someone had suddenly shoved Blu-Tack down them and he couldn't hear. 'Either I'm having the most bizarre dream in the world, or you just said you wanted a baby.' He pressed the plunger, poured out two steaming mugs of strong coffee, and pushed one towards me with a puzzled look.

I nodded. 'Yep, that's what I said.'

'But you said you never wanted kids.' His eyebrows furrowed together so he looked like he had a unibrow.

I laughed. A slight chuckle at first. Then it turned into a giggle, then side-splitting, hilarious, uncontrollable laughter. I slammed the table with my hand. 'I know! How weird is that? I've gone through my whole life being adamant I don't want kids. Not a maternal twinge in my body. Until today.'

He threw me a who-are-you-and-what-the-fuck-have-you-done-with-my-wife? kind of look.

7

'Gina, are you ill? Have you got a fever?' He reached out and touched my forehead.

'No. It's just the most bizarre thing. All of a sudden, the only thing I know is I want a baby. Your baby.' I reached forward and grabbed his hand, squeezing it. 'So, what do you think?' I jumped up from the chair and leapt onto his knee, wrapping my arms around his neck. 'It's a great idea, isn't it? You'd make a fantastic dad. Look how good you are with Jayne's kids.'

'Well, yeah. I mean, I guess I've always wanted to have kids one day. I just thought it would eventually happen when I was in my thirties.'

'You *are* in your thirties.' I grinned.

'Oh, God, you're right. When did that happen? In my head I'm still twenty-one.' He grinned back.

'So this is perfect timing,' I said. 'I mean, we can afford a baby now you're doing so well at work. We've got a three-bed house so it's big enough. I can still do my beauty business from home. And our kids would be adorable.' I clapped my hands together with excitement. 'Just think, they'd have your thick, dark hair, my green eyes, your calm-in-a-crisis, gentle nature, and my determination. What a perfect combination!'

'I need some caffeine to let this sink in.' He took a huge gulp of coffee, swallowing thoughtfully. 'I suppose they'd also have your dirty laugh, sense of humour, and fun-loving spirit. And they'd have both my practical ability to do DIY, and my business brain.'

'Oh, yeah, what else?' I grinned, getting into the swing of things. 'My organizational skills.'

'As long as they don't get your map-reading skills. They'll get lost on the way out of your womb if they do.' He chuckled.

'Or your leave-dirty-socks-around-the-house skills.' I raised an eyebrow. 'So, what do you think?' I looked down at him expectantly.

'Does that mean we can start trying now?' he raised a

8

seductive eyebrow at me.

I leapt off him and grabbed his hand, pulling him up. 'Hell, yeah!'

Sex, Sex, and More Sex

I'd been taking the pill ever since I was fifteen for heavy periods that felt like Freddy Krueger was trying to rip his way out of me, and since then I'd been as regular as my credit card bills. Every twenty-eight days, voila! I could almost time it down to the correct hour.

So the first month after I stopped taking it, when I didn't get my period at the allotted time, I thought, bloody hell, that was quick! I'm pregnant already. Out with the pill, nookie a couple of times a month, and hey presto – Mum's the word!

I rushed off to the chemist to buy a pregnancy test with a goofy grin plastered all over my face, grabbed the first one I saw, and zoomed back. Throwing my bag on the floor, I ran up the stairs to the bathroom like an Olympic-medal-winning hurdler and tore open the protective cellophane wrapper, ripping the box in my excitement.

I pulled out one of the two sticks, peeled off the outer foil, and was about to pee on it when I realized I had to actually read the instructions to make sure I was getting it right:

1) Wash your hands with soap and water before removing stick from foil wrapper.
Oh, crap, too late! Well, I only touched the holding end, not the bit you pee on, so that should be OK.
2) Remove testing stick from foil wrapping.
Yes, I know about that part.
3) Sit on toilet.
Well, duh! I'm not going to wee on it in the middle of the bathroom floor! Hurry up, get to the good bit.

4) Ensuring the stick is pointing downwards, urinate directly on the end of the plastic stick using a midstream sample.

What does that mean?

Note: Midstream sample means you should let out a bit of urine first, then collect the sample mid flow.

Right. Got it. I think. How do you know exactly when midstream is? It's not like I've got an invisible bladder wall I can see. This is getting complicated.

5) Urinate for 5 seconds only.

Easy peasy.

6) Place the test stick on a flat surface. You will see a line in the control window. (See figure 2.)

OK.

7) Read your results after 2 minutes. If you have two vertical blue lines in the test window, you are pregnant. If you have a single vertical line, you are not pregnant.

And I was off. Hopefully collecting midstream flow, although it wasn't until I'd finished my wee that I realized I was a bit on the early side, but I figured I was close enough.

Knickers and jeans pulled up, I stared at the stick with my heart threatening to explode out of my chest.

Maybe I shouldn't look at it. Was it the same as a watched kettle never boiling? Did a watched pregnancy test never shout PREGNANT! I gnawed on my lower lip and looked away, but as if by some kind of magnetic pull, I felt my neck pinging back round to stare at it.

I checked my watch.

One minute.

I tapped my nails along the sink. A faint blue line appeared in the test window.

Come on, come on. OK, maybe I should explain now that patience has never been my thing. I was even born early.

Right, not looking now.

I turned my back on it and stared at the wooden floorboards so hard my vision blurred.

I checked my watch again.

Two minutes.

Hurrah!

I swung back around and stared at the stick.

Bollocks, crap, fuck!

A single blue line. That meant I wasn't pregnant. Unless…

Unless I'd messed it up somehow. Yes, that was it. I'd messed it up. I'd need to use the other test stick to try again, but I was all weed out.

Damn.

Six glasses of water, forty-five minutes, and a test stick later, the result was the same.

So I wasn't pregnant this month, but that was OK. Whether it took one month or two months didn't really matter. I mean, it was going to be pretty easy to get pregnant, wasn't it? After all, when I was around fifteen my mum was always telling me how easy it was, and how I should make sure I used a condom, as well as the pill (in those days there wasn't so much info about STDs and safe sex, so the additional willy armour was only required to ward off unwanted sperm). And, if possible, she said I should use a chastity belt, too. According to Mum, you just had to touch a boy's bits and you'd get pregnant. That little saying was drummed into me constantly. And that's pretty much what the sex education teacher told us at school. Although now I know they were trying to scare our young, sexually active minds, which is a good thing, but honestly, how hard could it actually be to conceive? Millions of women around the world must be achieving it every second.

Karl breezed in from work that night and gave me a kiss on the cheek as I was in the converted garage that I used for my beauty business. 'Thank God it's Friday.' He tugged at his tie to loosen it. 'This week at work's been manic.'

Karl had recently been promoted to regional sales manager for Cussler Telecommunications, a company that supplied phone lines, internet, and satellite TV.

'So what shall we do tonight? Meet Amelia and Dan down

the pub or get a greasy Chinese takeaway with a bottle of wine?'

'Don't mind,' I sighed, busying myself as I tidied away wax applicators, nail varnish, and massage oil.

'You're quiet. What's up?' he said.

'I'm not pregnant.' I pulled a face at him.

He looked at me, an amused smile tugging at the corners of his lips. 'It's only been a month.' He held his arms open and I stepped into them.

'I know. But I was convinced I was pregnant because I was late. And those skinny jeans I bought last month were getting tight.' Although that could be from scoffing too many chocolate Hobnobs. Since our corner shop had a special offer on at the moment of buy one packet get one free, I'd kind of overindulged a smidgen. In my defence, I'd like to say that I'd thought it was a food craving at the time and perfectly acceptable, instead of downright gluttonous.

'It's not going to happen overnight.' Karl rested his chin on my head. 'So what if it takes a few months? It's not the end of the world. You'll see, this time next year we'll probably be celebrating Cecil's first birthday.'

'Cecil?' I snorted, managing a smile. 'We're not calling our kid Cecil!'

'Yeah, you're right. Cuthbert is much better. Or Tarquin.'

I gave him a playful punch to his arm. 'Esmerelda.'

'No way! Guinevere.'

'Marlene,' I giggled, then sighed into his shoulders. 'OK, you're right. So what if it takes a couple of months.'

'That's because I'm a man and we're always right.'

'Don't push it.'

'Anyway, we're both young and healthy. Probably all you need to do is relax and stop thinking about it, and it will just happen.'

'Well, that's easier said than done,' I huffed. 'And what if something's wrong?'

'Nothing's wrong! In fact, why don't we get a quickie in now to prove it?' He slid his warm hands up the back of my jumper, stroking his fingers up and down my spine.

'Ooh, I like your style!' I said as his fingers probed the underneath of my bra, and our clothes were suddenly a jumble on the floor. 'Wait!' I pulled apart before things got too heated. 'We need to do it where I can put my legs comfortably in the air afterwards.'

'What?'

'Well, I was talking to Amelia the other day and she told me her sister said you need to stick your legs in the air after sex so that the sperm has a better chance of swimming up your fallopian tubes.'

'You're going to do a handstand after we have sex?' he chuckled. 'Kinky! That puts a new slant on bedroom acrobatics.'

'And no oral sex anymore,' I said, pulling a disappointed face.

'For me or you?'

'Me. Apparently saliva can negatively affect sperm.' I tilted my head, thinking. 'On second thought, maybe you shouldn't have any, either, just to be on the safe side.'

'Damn.'

'Double damn.'

But deep down I couldn't shake the sneaking suspicion something wasn't all it was meant to be in fertility land. I knew the instructions on the pill said to always use additional contraception until you started your next month's dose if you were sick, had the squits, or accidentally missed one. In fifteen years, I'd had food poising several times (with both projectile vomiting and squits involved – a double whammy), I'd missed a lot more than one dose of it in all that time, and one month I'd even missed a whole two weeks' worth when Karl and I went on holiday and I forgot to pack them. And never once in all that time did I use a condom.

For the next six months we were having so much sex I thought his willy might actually fall off from overuse.

14

Lounge, kitchen, bedroom, hallway; plus an adventurous phase in empty fields and woods, which soon stopped when I ended up getting a tick on my bum. (That was highly embarrassing going to Accident and Emergency to get it removed, especially when the first doctor had never been faced with a bum-tick before and had to consult a plethora of doctors before I could finally get it extracted. And it was bloody painful!)

The only trouble was, the more we had sex, the more my periods were getting further and further apart. Sometimes it would be every two months, sometimes four, so I didn't have a clue when and if I was actually ovulating.

There was only one thing for it: the Internet. Google became my new best friend. Every spare chance I got I was on there looking up fertility stuff. Some of it blew my mind...

Cervical Mucus:

Cervical mucus is a good indicator that ovulation is about to take place. In order to maximise your chances of getting pregnant, timing intercourse around ovulation is essential. Your mucus lets you predict your most fertile time.

As you reach ovulation, your cervical mucus changes in consistency so that it is much more sperm-friendly. During your monthly cycle the mucus changes from dry and sticky, to creamy, to wet, to a raw egg white consistency, then back to dry and sticky again.

When it reaches the raw egg white stage ovulation is approaching. This is the most productive time to have sex.

You can check your mucus by inserting a clean finger into your vagina. If it is very wet and stretches between your fingers and resembles raw egg white, ovulation is just around the corner.

What the fuck! How had I been walking around for thirty-three years with egg white up my fufu and never even noticed? Did every other woman in the world know this

15

secret except me?

Basal Body Temperature:

Charting your Basal Body Temperature can determine if you've been missing the ideal time to get pregnant. Examples of charts can be found on fertilityfriend.co.uk.

Once you have a chart, you need to get a digital thermometer designed to measure your Basal Body Temperature.

1) You need to take it at the same time every morning (give or take 30 mins).

2) Very important! You need to take your temperature before you do anything else. You cannot walk around, sit up, drink, eat, talk. The minute you wake up, you need to put the thermometer in your mouth.

3) Very important! You need at least 3-4 hours constant sleep before taking your temperature. If you've had interrupted sleep, or a late night, it may make the results inaccurate.

4) Record your daily temperature on your chart.

Ideally, you should record your temperature throughout your entire cycle.

This method is a great way to see when and if you're ovulating, but it doesn't predict ovulation. Your BBT will only rise and remain higher after ovulation has taken place.

Ideally, you should make love every other day around ovulation.

OK, I got that. It kind of made sense. So all I needed was a thermometer and I was good to go.

Ovulation Predictor Kit:

There are only a few days in a woman's cycle when she can conceive. Ovulation Predictor Kits are used in the same way as a pregnancy test and work by detecting the Luteinising Hormone levels in your urine. When ovulation approaches, the LH levels spike, which is called an LH surge. Approximately 24-36 hours after the surge, ovulation takes place.

When you detect the surge, you will probably ovulate within 24 -48 hours. To maximise your chances of getting pregnant, you should ideally have sex within 24 hours of detection. Sperm can survive for 1-5 days, depending on conditions.

Omigod, this was getting harder and harder. I didn't know I only had two fertile days every cycle. How did anyone ever manage to get pregnant at that rate?

Female Biology:

When a woman is born, she has over 1 million eggs in her ovaries. By puberty, she'll only have around 300,000 left. Only 300 of these will mature and be released during her reproductive years.

Uh-oh, this is getting worse and worse. What was the point in having 1 million eggs when you're born if you're not going to use them then? How stupid was that? It was like winning the lottery but never being able to spend the money until you reached ninety. I stared at the screen as a sliver of dread danced down my spine. The chances of getting pregnant were getting slimmer and slimmer. Had my ovaries already shrivelled up like a couple of dried old prunes?

I switched the computer off then before I found out something even more depressing.

In between a pedicure on Mrs Omeroyd, whose feet looked like pigs' trotters, and a Brazilian wax on Stella, I rushed off to the chemist for supplies.

I spent an hour perusing the different kits and thermometers. Was one better than the other? Should I get a more expensive kit? How many would I need? Worst case scenario, if my period was coming every four months, I'd use around sixty strips per cycle.

I loaded up two boxes containing thirty per box and took everything to the checkout.

I nearly had a heart attack when the checkout girl said, 'Sixty pounds, please.'

'What are they made of? Gold?' I asked, handing over some crumpled notes. Still, I'd only need this lot. Now I had the tools to predict ovulation, I'd be pregnant in no time. Simple.

Green Tea and Baggy Boxers

I was shopping with my best friend Amelia in town just before Christmas, stocking up on last minute pressies, when I had my first proper freak-out moment about the lack of action on the baby front.

The shopping centre was swarming with mothers and children. Toddlers, teenagers, babies, everywhere I looked. I swallowed down a hard lump in my throat and blinked back tears as I pretended to be interested in Body Shop gift sets for Karl, socks (again) for Dad, and a new broomstick for my snooty stepmum, Lavinia.

Who cared about all that material stuff anymore? I knew what I wanted for Christmas, but it just wasn't happening. If I heard "Little Drummer Boy" blasting out of the shops sound system, along with all the other crappy Christmas songs, I wouldn't be responsible for my actions.

And why had all these calendar shops sprung up in every available empty space? All I'd done for the last eight months was chart things on calendars – daily body temperature, possible ovulation dates, egg white, when my bastarding period arrived, and how long my cycle was. I didn't need a bloody reminder, thanks very much! It was like fate was taunting me. What if I was in the same position this time next year?

'So what happened at the doctor's yesterday? Did you get the results of your blood tests?' Amelia asked as she perused a boxed set of beers for her husband, Dan.

'Yes.' I nodded glumly.

She glanced up with expectation, her hazel eyes fixing on

mine. 'Well, don't keep me in suspense. Is it good or bad?'

'Bad-ish.' I exhaled a deep sigh. I'd been taking my basal body temperature for six months now, and it was up and down more times than the price of petrol. Along with my irregular periods, and blood tests on days four and twenty-one of my cycle to check my hormone levels, it all confirmed I had an ovulatory dysfunction. 'I'm dysfunctional,' I said.

'Oh, Gina.' She put the beer back on the display shelf and wrapped me in a hug. 'But they can do something about it, right?' She pulled back, searching my face for signs of good news.

'I have to have some more tests done. A scan to see if I've got polycystic ovaries, and an HCG test to check if my fallopian tubes are OK. Then they're probably going to give me Clomid, which is some kind of drug to trigger ovulation.'

'And what's the success rate with it?'

'Apparently it can start ovulation in about eighty percent of women, and about forty percent of women get pregnant within six months of treatment,' I said.

'Well that's great, then.'

I nodded again and sniffed. I'd always been a glass is half-full kind of girl, but now I was starting to doubt everything. What if I fell into the sixty percent category who didn't get pregnant?

In the distance, I spied a cute baby girl in a buggy, dressed up in a reindeer outfit, complete with a reindeer headband that had waggly antlers poking out on springs. Her cheeks were pink from the stifling heat of the shop. As she threw a stuffed teddy bear out of her pram, giggling at it, her mum looked down at her with such an expression of pure love I had a sudden stabbing pain in my chest. I had to get out of there.

I pushed my way through the crowds to the entrance and leaned my back against the cold brick wall outside, taking deep gulps of air.

Amelia appeared by my side within seconds, a crinkled

frown on her face. 'It *will* work. I know it will, Gina.' She nodded so much her black bob escaped from being tucked behind her ears and fell forward, framing her face. 'You just have to be positive and relax. Stop thinking about it so much.'

Yes, but that was easy for everyone else to say. It was all right for her and Dan – they'd never wanted kids. They were perfectly happy together with no new additions to the family, instead doting on their three cats, and nieces and nephews that they were glad to "give back" to their parents at the end of the day. Why couldn't I be like that? Well, actually that was the old me. I was always adamant I never wanted kids. If any of our friends got pregnant in the past, Amelia and I used to have smug conversations about all the things we'd rather do than have kids...

Me: I'd rather have an affair with Gordon Brown than have kids.

Amelia: Or David Blunkett.

Me: Most definitely.

Amelia: All they do is poop and cry. I can't see the attraction. I'd rather get my leg chewed off by an alligator than change dirty nappies.

Me: I'd rather live on a desert island for a year with no wine than deal with screaming babies.

Amelia: And no chocolate.

Me: Yep. I'd rather have all my teeth extracted with no anaesthetic.

...But now maybe it was too late. My body clock was clanging in my ear with annoying persistence, and I couldn't help wondering what would've happened if we'd started trying sooner. I envied Amelia and Dan. I wished I could go back to those days, where it was just Karl and me, and the only thing I had to worry about was what to cook for dinner that night, which film we were going to watch, or which party we were going to. Now it just seemed like my brain was wired up wrong and all I could think about was getting pregnant. Even a simple shopping trip just rammed down my throat that I was still very un-pregnant.

'Oh, God, I forgot to give you this!' She rummaged around in her bag. 'I found this article in the newspaper the other day so I thought you should take a look.' She thrust it in my hand.

I tried to look at it but my eyes were blurry with tears.

'Here.' She handed me a tissue.

I glanced up and gave her a weak smile as I wiped my eyes. 'Thanks,' I said, ignoring the crowds who were busy rubbernecking at me as they walked past.

The article was written by a female nutritionist called Dr Julia Jones, who had lots of credits after her name, saying how diet was really important to aid fertility.

As I took in every word slowly, I read three women's success stories. One of them had been trying to get pregnant for six years, and after following Julia's advice, she fell pregnant within six months. Another woman had gone through three IVF treatments and had given up hope when she bought Julia's book and started implementing her recommended dietary changes, then she had twins within nine months. The last woman had been told by all the doctors she'd never have kids and got pregnant a year after following Julia's advice. The title of the book and website was listed at the end.

'Come on.' I grabbed Amelia's arm and dragged her towards the nearest bookshop with a new bounce in my step. This was it. All I had to do was change my diet and it would work.

Five hours later, I'd read the book cover to cover and was feeling more positive. If I followed her advice, I had a fantastic chance of getting pregnant. Dr Julia Jones didn't get to be a bestselling nutritionist by talking crap, or eating crap, for that matter, so what she says goes from now on. She would be my new healthy-eating guru. All I had to do was follow her advice:

Out with the caffeine; in with the green tea, peppermint tea, nettle tea (blah! Sounded gross. Who wanted to drink a cup of scratchy weeds?).

Sugar and refined carbs were not my friend, apparently. (Damn, chocolate was definitely my friend!) Whole-wheat grains and oats were recommended. (Right, so gloopy porridge for breakfast instead of Coco Pops. Yum. *Not.*)

Pulses like lentils and quinoa (never heard of it), were good sources of protein instead of meat.

Everything should be organic to reduce the amount of pesticides and hormones that could be messing up my system.

Fresh fruits and veggies were the name of the game.

Nuts (not Karl's for once) and fresh, oily fish were a must. (Ew, mackerel made me feel nauseous at just the whiff of it.)

Sodas, artificial sweeteners, and E numbers were worse than cyanide.

Plus, a list of vitamins, minerals to combat any deficiencies, and the herbal supplement Vitex, which was good for rebalancing hormone levels and normalizing ovulation.

Severely reducing, or cutting out alcohol completely (Not too keen on that part. I loved wine, but I wanted a baby more, so, I guess I'd have to do it.)

No problemo. I could do this!

As soon as Karl came home from a bike ride with Dan I said, 'We're going shopping,' with a huge smile on my face.

'Oh, God,' he groaned, sitting on the bottom step and pulling off his trainers. 'Haven't you been shopping all afternoon with Amelia? I bet it's murder out there with the Christmas rush.'

'No, we're going food shopping. To the supermarket.' I grabbed his coat and thrust it towards him.

He glanced down at his cycling shorts and sweaty top. 'I

23

need a bath first! I can't go out like this. And didn't you go food shopping the other day? We've got loads of stuff in the house.'

'Well, first of all, you can't have a hot bath anymore because it's bad for your sperm, and second, we have to stock up on loads of healthy food.' I filled him in on Julia's book. 'Oh, and after your lukewarm shower, not *bath,* you have to wear these.' I opened up a bag full of new baggy boxer shorts I'd bought in town after reading that tight ones can cause bollock asphyxiation and damage sperm.

He looked at me like I'd just suggested a threesome with a cyborg, then peered in the bag. 'Are you having a laugh?' He pulled out some oversized, baggy boxers that, OK, I admit, looked like something a seventy-year-old granddad would wear.

'If it helps increase those little swimmers, who cares? Practical, medical advice overrules vanity from now on. You've got to do the sperm test on Monday morning so I can take it to the hospital, and I want those little guys to pass with flying colours. At least it will be one less thing to worry about.'

'Do you know how uncomfortable these are going to be? I love my tighties, they keep me all compact and cosy. I'll be flopping around all over the place in these.' He put his hands in one of the short legs and pulled the material apart to see how wide it was. 'Fucking hell, I could fit a jumbo jet in one of these legs. You'll be buying me a kilt next.'

'Hey, great idea!' I made a mental note to order him one online. 'And you can't go cycling anymore.' I bit my lip, waiting for the next outburst. 'It constricts the blood flow to your nuts, apparently.'

'But I've been cycling for twenty years.' He threw up his hands in a defeated gesture. 'What *am* I allowed to do now?'

I just smiled sweetly. 'Come on, then, hurry up and get in the shower so we can go.'

'So what are we having for dinner?' Karl dumped the last

food-filled carrier bag on the kitchen worktop two hours later.

'Vegetarian shepherd's pie with spinach, lentils, red peppers, tomatoes and carrots, with a sweet potato topping, and a leafy green salad on the side. Then for an evening snack you can have pumpkin seeds.'

He pulled a horrified face, like I'd just suggested feeding him kangaroo's bollocks. (I had nuts on the brain!)

'They're all good for both your sperm and me,' I said, reading the instructions on the packet of dried lentils. Soak overnight before use, it said. Damn. I could see this was going to get complicated. 'Minus the lentils,' I added, thinking I could use them for something tomorrow, that was if I ever managed to get off the Internet because I'd be too busy looking up new recipes to make dinners with all this new stuff.

'Right. But please don't tell me I can't have a beer tonight. That's going to just about finish me off.'

'Er...I hate to break it to you but alcohol is out, too,' I said, thinking I could kill a glass of wine right about now. Or a bottle. I glanced over at the wine rack in the corner of the kitchen. A nice Chilean red was seriously calling my name.

No! Don't look at the wine. Focus. Wine's nice but a baby is better. Stop looking!

He followed my gaze. 'What about wine? Wine's OK, isn't it? Red wine's good for...' he tilted his head, looking like he was racking his brain to come up with something it was good for. 'Your heart!' he finally said, looking pretty pleased with himself.

'According to Julia, any alcohol negatively affects a woman's eggs, and it can increase oestrogen in males, which might interfere with sperm production. It's also a toxin that kills off sperm-generating cells in your nuts.' I threw a last longing look at the wine.

'So we have to turn into teetotal vegetarians to get pregnant, otherwise I'll end up with toxic nuts and manboobs?'

I gave him a sympathetic smile. 'That's about the size of it. Although, we can still have organic meat, but it's pretty expensive so we'll be having lots of healthy protein things like quinoa.' I slipped my arms around his neck and kissed him.

'I don't even think I want to know what that is.' He rested his chin on the top of my head and groaned. 'OK, babe. Anything I have to do to get our Cecil, I'll do.'

Just Relax!

'Come on, we're going to be late round your dad and Lavinia's,' Karl whispered while I was on the phone to Poppy.

I'd met Poppy online at the Fertility Friends website about a month before and we'd started messaging each other. Then it progressed to phone calls. From her profile picture on the website she looked like an original hippie. Tie-dye clothes, a silver hoop through her nose, and about a million on each ear, blonde dreadlocks.

'So Karl's got to do his sperm test tomorrow, and I'm having my scan and HCG test next week,' I told her.

'Well, that's good,' she said. 'At least you might get some more idea of where you are next week. But you really need to stop worrying so much about it and have some fun.'

I snorted. I was sick of people telling me that. It was like telling someone trying to give up smoking not to think about cigarettes. It just made you think about them even more.

Poppy laughed. 'I know, it's easier said than done, believe me. But if you constantly obsess about it, you're likely to self-sabotage.'

I frowned. 'Huh? What do you mean?'

'Well, you know when you really, desperately want something in life, it just never seems to happen, but when you're not that interested in something you seem to get it easily. It seems to just come to you without even trying.'

'Yes.'

'I think a lot of the time we self-sabotage when we desperately want something, because deep down we're afraid what will happen when we get it. If we don't care too much

27

about something, it doesn't matter whether we get it or not, but when we care deeply, there's a huge risk in getting it. What if it doesn't work out, will I be unhappy, then? What if I get it and I love it, but then it's taken away from me? What if I get it but there's another cost to having it – one I haven't thought of yet? What if I lose something else along the way in trying to find it? Do you see what I mean?' she asked.

'So you're saying we unconsciously put obstacles in the way of getting what we want because we're afraid of what will happen when we get it?' Wow, I'd never thought about it before. Did it make sense? I wracked my brains, trying to think back to things I'd really wanted in life. When I was younger, I wanted to be an astronaut and that didn't happen. What else? Oh, yes, there was the time in beauty school when I wanted to win the award for the best French manicure, but that didn't happen, which was a shame because the prize was a twenty-quid voucher for the cinema and I had a huge crush on Patrick Swayze who was starring in *Dirty Dancing* at the time.

'It could be because of your mum,' Poppy's voice interrupted my brain-searching as Karl paced up and down the kitchen, doing flapping hurry-up motions with his hands.

I glared at him and tuned back into Poppy. This was just getting interesting.

'Your mum died when you were seventeen, which was right about the time you were blossoming as a woman. Maybe you're worried that if you have a baby, somehow you'll be taken away from it, or it will be taken away from you, and so inadvertently your brain or body is putting obstacles in the way of getting pregnant.'

Oh, God, maybe she had a point. 'I've never heard of that before, but maybe you're right.'

'Your mind is a powerful tool. When you hear the phrase "mind over matter," it's true. Your subconscious actually holds more power than your conscious mind. Even though you're telling everyone that you want a baby, if you have a subconscious belief that it's unattainable, you're likely to be using yourself as an obstacle.'

I took a deep breath and let that sink in. Could she really be on to something about my mum? I mean, I was an only child so we were very close, and even now, I still felt the emptiness of not having her here. I knew she would understand what I was going through and be my rock of support. I guess seventeen is a pretty bad age to lose your mum, when you need to turn to her for guidance on relationships, broken hearts, new jobs, and generally flourishing into a woman. Could I really be self-sabotaging because I was scared of losing a baby somehow when I got it? Possibly. Did I have a really have a fear of succeeding in having a baby? A dread that somehow I might be a failure as a mum, or that he or she might be suddenly whipped away from me in the blink of an eye, like Mum? And if so, what could I do about it?

'OK, so what can I do to change that?' I said. 'If that is what's going on.'

'Well, acknowledging it is probably the first step. Maybe you should try and repeat some mantra every day to introduce positive thoughts.' She paused for a moment. 'Something like, "I can be happy as a mother," or "the past will not become the future." If you say it often enough, it might get through to your subconscious. I'd also recommend doing some relaxation CDs. There's a new one out especially for fertility that you can order,' she said as Karl poked me to hurry up.

I stuck my tongue out at him. 'OK, that's really helpful, Poppy, thanks. I'll think about what you said and get the CD.'

'And don't forget to call me any time.'

'Right back at ya!' I said and hung up.

'Come on, we're going to be late,' Karl said as I flung on my coat. 'I don't want to risk the wrath of Lavinia.'

I curled my lip up and groaned. Dad had met Lavinia six years ago, and she was the complete opposite of my mum. How can I describe her without sounding like a complete bitch? Hmm…Lavinia was the most difficult woman I'd ever met. Nothing was ever right for her, and she complained constantly about everything. God knows how Dad put up with her, although he was so placid, he probably just went along with her for a quiet life. Whereas mum had been full of fun and life and the kindest person I'd ever known, Lavinia was…well, a self-centred, snooty witch. But somehow, and I haven't got the foggiest idea how, she seemed to make Dad happy, so I vowed ages ago to be the perfect stepdaughter and not upset the applecart. Along with Lavinia came a stepsister called Jayne, who was pretty much the spitting image of Lavinia, in looks and personality. She was married to Wayne, and I still couldn't say Jayne and Wayne in the same sentence without chuckling to myself. OK, childish I know, but I couldn't help myself.

'Shit! I forgot to bring the wine!' I said as we pulled up outside their house across town.

'Good, it's not like we're drinking it anyway,' Karl said. 'I might be tempted to smack Lavinia over the head with it if it's in my reach. Well, after being tempted to drink the whole bottle.'

Since Karl's parents lived in Spain, we hardly ever got to see his side of the family, and even though he loved my dad like a second father figure, he felt the same about Lavinia as I did, tolerating her for Dad's sake.

'No, I'd bought some non-alcoholic elderflower wine to bring.' I opened their gate and walked up the driveway.

'Yum.' He gave me a look that said it sounded anything but yum.

'Lavinia will be in moany mode now. Why don't you nip down to the corner shop and grab a bottle?' I said. 'I'll just have water.'

'OK.' He kissed the top of my nose as I rang the doorbell, probably grateful for a few more minutes of non-Lavinia time.

Oh, and speak of the devil…she swung open the door and gave me a tight smile. 'Gina, how lovely of you to make it.'

She glanced at my empty, non-wine bearing hands and her mouth pinched slightly. 'Come in.' She stepped back and let me enter.

'So how've you been?' I asked as she closed the door.

'Wonderful, thanks. Everyone's in the lounge.' She disappeared as I slipped off my coat and hung it on the hook by the door.

Well, I'm good, too, thanks for asking!

'Aunty Gina!' Rupert and Quentin, Jayne and Wayne's (ha ha!) two sons came bounding over to hug me.

Rupert was seven and hugged me tight around the waist, resting his head on my stomach and gazing up at me like a long-lost friend. Quentin was nine and nestled his head into me until I put my arm around him. I kissed the tops of their heads. They smelt of grass and toothpaste.

'How are you both?' I said, smiling down at them.

'Now, now, boys, let Gina go.' Jayne clapped her hands to get their attention like they were a couple of dogs she was trying to distract. 'I'm sure she doesn't want to be hassled by you as soon as she walks in the door.'

'Of course I do!' I said, ruffling their hair. 'What have you been up to? How's school? How's the football team going?' I asked them.

'Do you want to see the drawing I did?' Rupert asked, pulling me towards the coffee table.

'No, Aunty Gina wants to see the new model dinosaur I made.' Quentin pulled me in the opposite direction.

'Boys, go outside and play,' Wayne barked at them. 'This is adult time now.'

They both screwed up their faces. 'Awwwwww, we want to play with Aunty Gina.'

Lavinia clapped her hands together briskly (like mother like daughter). 'Off you go, before you make a mess in here,' she said to them.

'OK, I promise to play Monopoly with you after dinner.' I winked at them and they gave me an excited thumbs-up before disappearing.

It was the same every time I saw them. Jayne and Wayne were both barristers with a thriving practice in London, and never seemed to have any time for their children. An endless round of live-in au pairs looked after them most of the time.

'Gina!' Dad entered the room with an apron round his waist that said *Top Chef* on it. He loved to cook, and I'd bought if for him for Christmas last year, although if I were married to Lavinia, I'd spend most of the time away from her in the kitchen, too. It was Dad's little haven since she never even made so much as a cup of tea. He crushed me in a hug. 'How are you? Any news on the baby front?' He pulled back, searching my face for good news.

I shook my head, determined for once not to get upset about it.

'Jayne got pregnant instantly both times,' Lavinia butted in. 'Didn't you?' She glanced over at Jayne who nodded with a smug smile on her face. 'I must say it runs in the family.' Lavinia propped herself on the edge of the sofa that had perfectly arranged and plumped cushions, smoothing her tight black pencil skirt over her knee. 'All our side are incredibly fertile.'

I fought the urge to growl at her. Or worse, batter her over the head with…I searched the room for battering equipment…the Monopoly board would do for starters.

Jayne guffawed. 'I just had to look at Wayne and I got pregnant. Both times.'

Yeah, hilarious!

'Oh, well.' Lavinia waved her hand. 'If you just stop worrying about it and relax, it will happen.'

OK, I think I let out a slight growl at that.

Dad pulled me tighter in a supportive embrace. At least he seemed to get it. 'Dinner will be ready in five minutes.' He thankfully changed the subject before dashing off back to the kitchen because something smelt of burning.

'Oh, I do hope you don't burn the roast potatoes again,' Lavinia called after Dad.

'I like them crispy,' I said, coming to Dad's defence.

'Cripsy? They were cremated.' Lavinia sighed. 'Where's Karl? He hasn't left you, has he?' she asked me. 'One of my friends ended up a neurotic mess when she was trying to have a baby. She split up with her husband because of it. I hope you're not moping around, getting all moody. That would be enough to put anyone off.'

I narrowed my eyes at her but she carried on anyway.

'I bet you're neglecting Karl. You need to make sure your house is always clean and tidy,' she said, glancing around her perfect show house, with not even a stray cauldron lying around, a satisfied smile on her face. 'You're a bit lacking in the housework department, after all. And talk to him about his work. Karl's career is very important to him. You don't want him to feel neglected because of all this baby business.' The way she said "baby business" came out sounding like a swear word.

I tried to drown out her "Life According to Lavinia" speech, but she was still droning on.

'You need to cook him some decent meals, too. The way to man's heart is through his stomach.' She gave me a condescending look, seeming to forget that she did no cooking whatsoever.

'Actually, I think the way to a man's heart is a bit lower than his stomach,' I said.

'Lavinia, can you get the door while I dish up?' Dad's voice rang out from the kitchen.

Lavinia sprang up from the seat like a cougar ready to pounce and marched to the front door to let Karl in, thankfully saving me from yet another rant.

'Where are the boys?' Karl asked Jayne and Wayne (he-he!) after he'd said his hellos.

'Outside so they don't disturb us,' Jayne said, flicking through a *House & Home* magazine. 'Honestly, I don't know why you want children. They're so demanding. You never get any time for yourself anymore. I'd love a moment's peace.'

Wayne nodded at his wife. 'It's not easy juggling high

profile criminal cases and having kids.'

'You're right, darling.' She patted his hand.

Karl and I exchanged a disbelieving look. Then I glanced out of the French doors into the garden and watched Rupert and Quentin tearing around, pretending to be planes, grinning from ear to ear and making engine noises. Why didn't their parents know how lucky they were? They had two precious, healthy boys who, despite their disinterested mum and dad, were turning out to be thoughtful, happy, and contented.

Normally I'd just let them get on with their ridiculous, selfish drivel, and maybe it was the caffeine and chocolate withdrawal kicking in, but I felt a hot angry flush crawling up my neck. 'So why did you have them, then, Jayne?' I demanded. 'I mean, I know they must've upset your busy work routine and social life and all that, so why bother?'

She carried on flicking through the magazine, oblivious to the edge in my tone. 'Do you know, I do ask myself that sometimes. When you have them, it's like you're trapped. No more relaxing holidays in the sun, no more quiet Sunday mornings with the papers. No more time to yourself without someone calling "Mum" every two minutes. It's exhausting!'

I stared at her for a second, not quite believing what she'd said. Then I turned on my heels and stormed into the steamy hot kitchen before I exploded and said something I'd regret.

Dinner wasn't much better, although luckily Dad steered the conversation away from babies and children. That was Dad – always the peacemaker.

Afterwards, Karl and I disappeared into the garden to play with the boys, and Dad brought out a green tea for me and a glass of non-alcoholic beer he'd found in the back of the cupboard for Karl.

Karl's eyes lit up. 'Beer!'

'Yes, but it's only pretend beer,' I said.

Karl took a huge gulp. 'I don't care. I can almost imagine it's the real thing.' He set it down on the patio table and I walked with Dad to a bench at the end of the garden where we could watch him playing football with Rupert and Quentin.

Dad sat down next to me and squeezed my hand. 'I know they can be a bit difficult sometimes, but they mean well,' he said, referring to the Lavinia tribe.

I seriously doubted it but I was too worn out to say anything.

'Your mum had trouble conceiving you, too,' he said.

My head whipped around to face him. 'Did she? I didn't know that. What happened?'

He smiled at me. 'You took two years to arrive. She had three miscarriages but the doctors couldn't find anything wrong with either of us.' He shrugged. 'It just took a bit of time, that's all. Try not to worry, love. I'm sure it will happen soon.' He patted my hand.

70-Mile-an-Hour-Sperm

'You need to have a wank now before you go to work,' I said to Karl as he had breakfast the next morning.

'Well, that will be a welcome change,' he said. 'One minute you're telling me I can't masturbate, now you're telling me I can.'

'Too much ejaculation around our fertile time can reduce the sperm quality so we need to keep your sperm for the essential days, but this is essential masturbation so you can break the previous no-wanking rule.' I thrust a small sample bottle I'd got from the doctors into his hand.

He took it, chewing thoughtfully on his toast. 'Why have you got your coat on?'

'The sperm only stays viable for up to two hours before it starts to deteriorate. As soon as you do it I need to rush up to the hospital so they can test it.'

'But we only live half an hour away from it.'

'What if there's a car accident, or I get car-jacked?' I said. I was sure he let out a small sigh but I carried on. 'What? It could happen! It happens all the time in South Africa.'

'We're not in bloody South Africa!' he said, and this time I definitely heard a sound. Something like a cross between a snort and a cough. 'What, do you think there's a female gang of pregnant wannabes lurking out there stealing sperm?'

I ignored his sarcastic outburst. '*And* it's rush hour,' I said. 'Do you want a hand?'

'Well, you standing there in your coat, tapping your foot, isn't exactly going to do it for me, is it? It's pretty hard to relax when I feel like I'm under pressure to perform all the time. I'm not a stud horse.'

36

OK, so maybe I was being an ickle tiny bit impatient, but all he had to do was ejaculate in a cup and that was his job done. How easy was that? He'd been masturbating probably since he was about twelve, what was the big deal? I had to go through all those other tests and possible hormone-induced hysteria, and the thought of what they might find was stressing me out. How selfish of him to get annoyed about having a bloody orgasm.

'Well, do it yourself, then,' I huffed.

'I will!' he stormed past me and disappeared up the stairs.

Twenty minutes later, as he sauntered down the stairs I rushed up to meet him, grabbing the test bottle like a relay sprinter handing over the baton, and shoving it down the front of my jeans.

'What are you doing?' He looked at me like I'd completely lost the plot.

'It has to be kept at body temperature so I'm keeping it down here for safety.' I shot out the door and slid behind the wheel of my sporty Volkswagen.

Ouch!

The plastic specimen pot jabbed me in the stomach. I readjusted it slightly and reversed out of the drive onto the main road, narrowly missing an oncoming bus.

OK, calm down, the hospital's not that far. It won't do to get killed by a bus on the way, the sensible part of my brain said.

Yes, but what if there's an unexpected accident on the motorway and all the cars get diverted through town? It would be gridlock. What if the car breaks down? What if there are roadworks? the neurotic part of my brain shouted at me.

I listened to the neurotic part and chugged off down the road past the school where all the mothers had parked up to drop off their kids, blocking the road and causing a huge traffic jam.

Come on, come on! I tapped on the dashboard, inching my way through the few spaces that opened up in the road as

37

cars coming from the opposite side pushed in.

I glanced at the clock on the dashboard. Fifteen minutes had passed. OK, still within time but, 'Hurry up!' I yelled at no one in particular.

Five minutes later, I managed to squeeze through a small gap, although it was touch and go whether I'd lose a wing mirror or not, and I made it to the end of the road that led to a dual carriageway. Rush hour traffic was in full swing and turning onto it proved to be a nightmare. No one would let me out, and the vehicles were speeding past as everyone was in Monday-morning-I'm-going-to-be-late-for-work panic mode.

After waiting exactly seven minutes and forty-five seconds (I couldn't help checking the clock) I managed to pull out on to the road, but by then the traffic was backed up for miles.

At a pace that would've won the national snail-racing championship, I then covered a mile in half an hour.

Damn, damn, damn. I had one hour, eight minutes and fifteen seconds left to get to the hospital. The traffic was still backed up, and at this rate, I wouldn't make it.

I shifted impatiently in my seat, glancing around frantically at the long queue of cars. I'd be stuck here forever, unless…I spied a farmer's field to my left with a tractor bumping along a dusty track in the middle of it. If I could get through the field, it would cut out all this traffic and I'd still be in with a chance.

Right. Here we go.

I swerved the steering wheel to the left, drove through a metal gate onto the track, and headed down a grassy embankment. Gripping the steering wheel tight, I bounced over dried mud and rocks, leaving a trail of billowing dust behind me. I ignored the crashing sounds as they hit the underside of the car. No time to think about any possible damage now.

Up in the distance the tractor had stopped. As I got nearer to it, the farmer jumped out and shrugged at me, arms wide, in a "what-the-hell-are-you-doing-driving-in-my-field?

gesture.

I wound the window down. 'Sorry! It's an emergency!' I gave him my best smile and bumbled past, heading towards the exit gate and back onto a main road.

One quick acceleration up another embankment and I managed to join a roundabout, where most of the traffic that I'd just missed was turning off onto the motorway. I swung a left onto another dual carriageway, which was relatively traffic-free and floored the accelerator down the road, ignoring my increasing speedometer.

Then I heard a siren behind me, and saw a police car swinging out of a side turning in my rearview mirror.

'Oh, great!' Just what I needed.

The police car flashed its lights for me to pull over.

I stopped the car, rummaging around in the glove box for my documents. In my haste to find them, a long, slim, glittery pink lip gloss came flying out into the footwell.

By then, a middle-aged policeman with salt and pepper hair stood by my door, knocking on the window with a stern expression.

'Just a sec!' I said, momentarily abandoning the search so I could open my window. 'Hello, officer, I'm just looking for my vehicle documents.' I turned back to the dashboard and snared the slim wallet. Aha! I grabbed it, and as I pulled it out, my insurance, tax, driving licence, and MOT all came flying out the end of it, landing in a jumbled mess next to the lip gloss.

'Oh, God,' I groaned. *Why me? Why is this happening to me?* 'Er…sorry.' I glanced up at him as he carefully studied every move I made.

'In a hurry are you, madam?'

'Well, kind of.' I gave him a slight smile.

'Do you know you were doing seventy in a fifty-mile-an-hour zone?'

'Sorry, officer. I wasn't aware of that,' I fibbed. I know, lying to the police would probably send me straight to criminal hell but I needed to get a move on. 'Can you just give me a ticket and I'll be on my way?'

He shifted his weight to the balls of his feet and back again before raising an eyebrow. 'Did I hear you correctly, madam? You actually want a ticket?'

'Yes.' *And hurry up about it!* I managed to retrieve the documents from the floor and pushed them through the window towards him. 'I'd like a ticket, please,' I said breathlessly, my eyes straying to the clock. I had an hour left.

He looked down at the documents but didn't examine them. 'No one has ever actually asked for a ticket before. In fact, most people will do anything *not* to get a ticket.' His voice took on an incredibly suspicious tone.

'Right, well, I'd love a ticket, please, officer. So if you could give me one I'd really appreciate it. Then I'll get out of your hair and you can get onto much more important enforcement thingyish stuff.'

He narrowed his eyes at me. 'Are you saying that speeding vehicles aren't important?'

'No!' I cried. 'Of course I wasn't suggesting that at all, officer. They're extremely important. Extremely,' I added again for emphasis.

'Do you know that most traffic accidents could be avoided if people adhered to the correct speed limit?

'Er...yes, I'm sure you're right. Could I have my ticket, please?'

'He leaned closer, peering over me to the inside of the car. 'Have you been drinking this morning, madam?'

'What? Of course not! It's only nine eighteen and fifteen seconds!'

'Would you get out of the vehicle, please?' He stepped back so I could swing the door open.

Oh, shit. How long was this going to take?

I got out and stood in front of him, silently willing him to get a move on.

'Have you got any offensive weapons in the car?'

'Pardon?' I thought I'd misheard him. Did I look like the

kind of person who carried around offensive weapons?

He pointed at the lip gloss lying in the footwell. 'What's that?'

What did he think I was going to do with it? Assault someone with a deadly lip gloss? Glitter them to death? 'That's lip gloss.'

'Let me see it.' He eyed me warily.

I reached into the car to retrieve it.

'Nice and slowly. I want to see your hands at all times.' He manoeuvred around the front of the vehicle so he could see me through the windscreen. 'We've had a spate of females assaulting people with pink screwdrivers, lately. You wouldn't happen to know anything about that, would you?' He narrowed his eyes at me.

'Of course not! I'm a respectable beauty therapist!' In super-slow motion I picked up the lip gloss and held it up, showing it to him through the window.

'Unscrew it so I can see what's inside.' He glared at me like I was a potential screwdriver assaulter.

I obliged, unscrewing the lid and waving the little foam wand at him. 'See? It's just lip gloss.'

'Hmm.' He raised an eyebrow. 'OK, out of the car, please.'

I got back out, maintaining my sloth-like speed in case any sudden movement could be interpreted wrongly and land me in handcuffs.

He leafed through my documents, taking his time, and I resisted the urge to tap my foot. Then he looked down at me, his eyes straying to the top of my jeans.

'What are you concealing down there?' His hand reached towards his belt, resting over his CS gas spray.

'Nothing.' My gaze shot to the top of my jeans. Where I'd been sitting down in the car, the white top of the specimen bottle had now wormed its way up and was visibly poking out of my waistband.

'Nice and slowly, I want to see you remove that item. And I don't want to see any sudden moves.' He unclipped the CS gas and held it in his outstretched hand in easy squirting range.

'Honestly, it's nothing. Well, OK, it's not nothing, obviously it's something, but it's not a weapon or anything, or drugs, or anything like that,' I babbled. 'Don't spray me. I have to get to the hospital.'

'I'll say it once again,' he said, eyeing my waistband like I was about to whip a Kalashnikov out of my knickers and annihilate everyone in a ten mile radius. 'Nice and slowly, let me see it.'

'OK, OK!' I clasped the bottle and pulled it out, practically shoving it in his face for him to inspect. 'But please don't make me keep it out in the cold air for too long; it has to be kept at body temperature.'

He squinted, peering at the contents. 'What is that?'

'Sperm. You see my husband and I are trying for a baby and I need to get it to the hospital really quickly. Oh, God, please don't arrest me. You don't know how long all this stuff takes. Every single month I'm waiting to get pregnant, and the doctors won't do anything until it's been at least six months, then you have to wait for all sorts of tests, and then before you know it another month has gone by and–'

He put his hand up to stop me, his eyes suddenly avoiding the sperm bottle. 'OK, OK! Why didn't you just tell me what was going on in the first place?'

I hung my head in shame. 'Because I was embarrassed to be carrying a pot of sperm down my knickers. You probably would've thought I was a complete lunatic, and it's not as if I like discussing the fact that I'm a sad excuse for a woman who can't get pregnant with all and sundry.'

He gave me a pitying look. 'I know what you're going through. My wife and I tried for three years before she got pregnant.' He nodded towards the pot. 'How much time have you got left before you need to get it there?'

I glanced at my watch and groaned. 'Fifteen minutes.'

'Right. I'll give you an escort. Let's go.' He rushed back to his car and turned on the lights and siren as I got into the

VW and cranked the engine.

He pulled out in front of me and I sat practically on his bumper the whole way there. I grabbed a parking space with five minutes to spare and legged it all the way to the pathology lab.

'Hello,' I said breathlessly to the lady behind the reception desk. 'I've got some sperm for you but it's nearly at the two-hour-old mark.'

'No problem, dear. I'll make sure they get to it straight away. Have you got the form from your doctor?'

'Yes.' I smiled gratefully, pushing the sample bottle and the form over the counter.

'Is that enough?' I said, eyeing the tube. It only looked like a tiny bit of sperm to me. What if they needed more? I didn't relish the thought of going through all this again.

'Oh, yes. The normal ejaculation is around half a teaspoon. This will be fine.' She wrapped the form around the sample and stood up. 'Check back with your doctor in about a week and the results should be there.'

I clutched my chest with relief. 'Thanks so much.'

My Womb is a Flower

I finished a gruelling pedicure on Mrs Omeroyd. Her bunions and ingrowing toenails were almost enough to distract me from thoughts of babies for a while. Almost, but not quite. I started fantasizing about what my baby's feet would look like. Would they have Karl's really hairy toes? Ew, I hoped not. If it was a girl, she wouldn't be too impressed. Would it have a long second toe, like me? I was always really embarrassed that it was longer than my big toe, but I'd read somewhere that it meant you were a fast runner, although that didn't ring true. I even used to come last in the egg and spoon race at junior school.

The post arrived when she'd left and, hurrah, my relaxation CD had come. I glanced at my watch. Perfect. I had two hours before my next client.

Poppy had told me the CD was fantastic for de-stressing and becoming one with your womb. I didn't know exactly what that entailed, and it sounded a bit scary to me, but I ordered it straight away off the Internet. For ten pounds, I couldn't go wrong. And if it worked, then woo hoo! I had a good feeling about it as I plopped it in the CD player next to our wooden six-foot bed and closed my eyes. This was exactly what I needed to relax me. I mean, it really wound me up when people told me to just stop thinking about getting pregnant and it would happen naturally. That's the worst thing you can say to someone who's been trying for so long. It made me want to scratch their eyes out. It's not like I *wanted* to think about it all the time. It's just some bizarre, unexplainable presence in my head that won't go away. This deep-seated, uncontrollable need to have Karl's baby. And anyway, I did stop thinking about it sometimes. Like when I was asleep.

'Close your eyes and imagine you are lying on a sandy beach,' a woman's gentle voice broke into my thoughts as the CD began.

OK, yes, I can do that.

'Let your legs and arms relax to the sides, palms facing upwards, as you sink into the warm, soft sand.'

Hey, I was way ahead of her.

'Feel the sand cushioning your body as you take deep breaths in and out. Feel the rhythmic sounds of the sea lapping at the shore. In and out,' she carried on for a few minutes with the in and out bit just to make sure I'd got the hang of it as I nestled into the bed – I mean, sand.

'Feel the stillness and calmness entering your body with every breath in, and feel the anxiety disappear with every breath out. Concentrate only on your breathing. Let it flow easily.'

Mmmm, lovely. Any minute now I'll be asleep. Maybe that's the idea – that it worked on your subconscious when you were asleep by thought projection. I'm sure I read somewhere about someone who learned Japanese by falling asleep to a CD. And that will definitely help if my subconscious really is into self-sabotage like Poppy thinks. Yes, the mind is a funny machine, isn't it? I saw on the news once about people who got terminal illnesses but suddenly managed to get well again through mind over matter.

'Free your mind from all its thoughts,' she carried on.

Right. Zip it, brain. I'm not thinking now.

'Imagine a bright, hot, white light entering your body from the tips of your toes, slowly working its way up to your womb. The light is nourishing and powerful. It will give your womb vitality and strength and nourishment, and will allow you to carry your baby safely. Silently repeat after me, "My womb is the centre of my being. It is capable of carrying a healthy embryo."'

I silently repeated it. *OK, it's a bit New Age-ish but never mind. Ha! Take that subconscious!*

'Now imagine the light touching your ovaries.'

Wait a sec, what does she mean by touching? Stroking? Tickling? Caressing? I don't want to get it wrong and blow them up with the light by accident.

'Don't forget to keep breathing. Deep, relaxing, soothing breaths.'

But what about the light? What am I supposed to do with it?

'Now imagine the light encapsulating your whole body, warming it. Your whole being is vitalised by the light. Repeat after me, I am the light. I feel the light. The light is power.'

Damn, I missed the ovaries. Does that matter? Won't it work now? I quickly repeated it before she could move on somewhere else.

'The light is fluttering down to your vagina.' For some reason she barked out the word "*vagina*" so it echoed around the room.

Ew…I hate that word. I cringed. It reminded me of a giant abyss. I suddenly imagined my fufu as a big, black, unaccommodating hole and that just did it for me. There was no bloody way this was going to work.

I jumped off the bed and jabbed the *off* button as tears sprang into my eyes. What a ridiculous idea, anyway. How stupid of me to even think a relaxation CD would help get me pregnant. Bloody Poppy. Bloody fertility treatment. And bloody VAGINA!

When Poppy rang to ask if I'd got the CD yet. I broke it to her gently that it didn't have the desired relaxation effect.

'OK, well, not to worry,' she said, her voice as upbeat and positive as ever. 'Sometimes I just make up my own mantras to use with relaxation. Why don't you just try saying something like, "My womb is a flower," or "Fertilize my egg," over and over again while you take deep breaths and close your eyes.'

Hmm…I couldn't see that working, either. 'OK,' I said.

'What you need to do is project positive thoughts to the Universe. It will help you receive cosmic enlightenment, and get rid of any negative energy surrounding you. I think your chakras are probably blocked, too.'

Oh, God, that didn't sound good. On the eve of my test to check if my fallopian tubes were clear, I didn't want to be hearing about any possible blockages.

'What does that mean, exactly? Is it like having a blocked nose, or something, and I can just take Beechams Powders to unblock them?' I chewed on my lip, waiting for her answer.

She chuckled. 'Not exactly. All of us have energy fields in us which are our chakras. If they're blocked for some reason, it can affect our mental and physical well-being. Positive thoughts can be a great way to unblock them.'

So as I lay in bed that night, thoughts whirring around in my brain like an out of control computer processor, I thought about what Poppy had said. Maybe she was right. I mean, it sounded a bit I've-had-too-many-acid-drops hippie stuff and all that, but what did I have to lose by asking the Universe for help? I decided to call the Universe Zelda, because it sounded like a Universe-ish kind of name, and I suspected she was a woman.

As Karl snored softly next to me I tried to block out all noises and closed my eyes, taking long, slow, deep breaths.

My womb is a flower, my womb is a flower, my womb is a flower. I silently repeated the mantra in my head, trying not to laugh.

What is that supposed to do, anyway?

Oh, shut up, brain!

OK, shutting up now. Come on subconscious, wake up!

I mean, really. Why a flower?

Zelda, my womb is a flower, OK?

Flowers are nice, though. Pretty. Unless you count the flowers on stinging nettles and then they're pretty pointless, aren't they? I mean, what's the reason for having flowers on

47

stinging nettles? What boyfriend in the world would buy a bunch of stinging nettles for their girlfriend as a nice Valentine's Day gift? Oh, actually, there was Craig who I dumped when I was about sixteen and he turned up on my doorstep the next day with a bunch for me.

Shut up, brain!

OK, OK!

Flowers are a sign of spring, rebirth, new beginnings. Yes, that's it! Birth.

Another deep breath in.

My womb is a flower. My womb is a flower.

And as I drifted off to sleep I repeated it over and over again.

Aghhhhhhhhhhhhhhhh!

That night I dreamt I gave birth to an onion. It was so vivid, as well. I was in the delivery suite, huffing and puffing away, and Karl was standing next to me with a happy grin on his face, mopping my sweating brow and gripping my hand as he looked lovingly into my eyes. In my dream, I could actually feel the onion coming out of my fufu.

I glanced down, exhausted but ecstatic, for the first glimpse of my beautiful baby. The doctor wrapped it up in a soft, fluffy blue blanket and handed it to me.

When I saw it was an onion, I screamed my head off. Then I woke up.

What the hell was that supposed to mean?

I was so freaked out I had to look up the meaning of dreams on the internet...

Seeing an onion in your dreams represents jealousy and envy from others if you're successful. (No, that couldn't be it. I didn't think any of my friends were jealous of me. I mean, Amelia didn't want a baby, and Kerry was a single career-girl who was perfectly happy with no kids.)

I kept looking...

If you dream of onions, you will go through a period of sorrow. (Yikes! I didn't like the sound of that one.)

Onions in dreams: You need to cry or get in touch with your emotional side. (What? I'd been crying enough tears every month when I didn't get pregnant to fill the Thames!)

Spiritual meaning of onions in dreams: The multi-layered aspect of the onion symbolizes the Cosmos – either the Universe or a personal journey. You need to look behind the obvious as you peel away the layers of the onion to achieve personal growth by working through your issues and getting closer to root causes. (Aha! Finally! I liked this definition better!)

So, Zelda had answered me. I had to go through some personal journey to get pregnant. And my tests were today so I really would be getting closer to the root causes of my problems. Maybe she was telling me not to worry, that everything would work out OK in the end.

A smile of satisfaction formed.

Yes, that was it. Absolutely.

We'd decided to go private to pay for the tests rather than endure the eight-month waiting list to get them done on the National Health Service. Time was speeding by, and at this rate I'd be seventy before I managed to get pregnant. I'd already had to wait until early in my next cycle to have it done so they could see if I was ovulating or not.

I had to have a full bladder for the ultrasound scan, and boy was it full. Maybe I'd overdone it on the water, but then I didn't have a clue how long it took to get from my stomach to my bladder. It wasn't something I normally thought about. Ooh, if they didn't hurry up, it wasn't going to be a pretty sight.

I crossed my legs. *Ah, big mistake!* I could hear my bladder screaming at me in pain. I quickly uncrossed them and moved around in my seat, trying to get into a position where I didn't want to wet myself. The only spot of good news was that trying to concentrate on keeping it in was stopping me from worrying about the tests.

'Gina,' a short and very round nurse called my name.

I took a deep breath and waddled towards her like John

Wayne to avoid any unnecessary spillage.

She smiled. 'I see you have a full bladder.'

'Full is an understatement.' I pulled a face.

'Follow me. The scan won't take long.' She led me into a small room with an examination couch and a couple of ultrasound machines on wheels. 'Take off your knickers and put the blanket over you. I'll be back with the gynaecologist in a moment.'

I did as she said, stepping up onto the couch like a geriatric in case my bladder popped.

I fidgeted for what felt like an eternity in bladder-squashing hell until she came back with the doctor, who was about fifty and balding. Why were most gynaecologists men? I wondered what he told his wife when they discussed his day at work over dinner. "Oh, yes, darling, I had a great day looking up a variety of lady gardens." I'm pretty sure his wife wouldn't be too impressed as she was tucking into her fufu-looking oysters when he discussed everything from the young, manicured topiary to the old, overgrown wild orchard he'd seen that day. Ew, it didn't bear thinking about.

'Right then, Gina. I'm Doctor Dye.' He fiddled around with the equipment, making sure it was on.

Er, hang on. Did he just say Doctor Die? A cold chill slammed through my veins. That was a bad sign if ever I saw one.

'Um…pardon?' I squeaked.

He turned back to me with a huge smile on his face. 'No, it's not spelt D-I-E. It's D-Y-E. Don't worry,' he chuckled, 'you're quite safe. I haven't lost a patient yet.'

'Right. Well, OK.' Although I wasn't entirely enthralled by it. What if Zelda was trying to tell me something?

'Just relax.' He rubbed some cold gel on my stomach.

Yeah, right. With Doctor Dye! He probably wouldn't even see my ovaries now. They were probably shrinking into my body this very second because he'd scared the shit out of them.

The nurse put a hand on my arm and gave me a reassuring

smile.

'OK, here we go.' He moved the head of the scanner over my abdomen as he faced the monitor. It was turned partially away from me so I could only see a bit of the screen.

Visions of my dream popped into my head.

'Now, you should be on about day eleven of your cycle, is that right?' he asked.

'Yes.' I craned my neck to see the screen he was looking at. But all I could make out were black and white lumps and blobby bits. Was that good or bad?

He moved the scanner head into various positions, pausing periodically to click something on the machine and take pictures, frowning occasionally.

Uh-oh, why was he frowning? My heart rate raced as I imagined all sorts of possible scenarios. Ovarian cancer, cysts, fibroids, an onion.

'Well, this is your uterus.' He pointed to some black and white shape on the screen that looked like a squid to me. 'It looks absolutely fine. No abnormalities, so that's good.'

I let out a breath of relief that I didn't even know I'd been holding.

'There are no fibroids or cysts, and you don't have polycystic ovaries, which is good news, too.'

'Great!' I smiled enthusiastically.

'But…'

Oh, crapping hell! I just knew there was going to be a but in there somewhere. My smile faded.

'I should see signs of follicles appearing by now, but I can't, which means you're not about to ovulate soon,' he said. 'Are your periods regular?'

'No. They can be anything from two months to four months apart.'

He moved the scanner around more, pressing on my stomach as my bladder made protest groans.

Ouch! Ouch, ouch, ouch. *I'm going to wet myself in a minute! Hurry up, hurry up!*

And then he said, 'OK, all done.'

Need a wee. Need a wee.

He removed the scanner and cleaned the head. 'There's a toilet through there. If you empty your bladder and come back, I'll do a transvaginal scan, too.' He pointed to a side door in the cubicle and I rushed off with the blanket clutched around me like my feet were on fire.

I plopped down onto the toilet as the waterworks started, sounding like Niagara Falls being let loose.

Oh, the relief!

Five times I thought I'd finished and each time there was still more. Where was it all coming from? My poor bladder had probably been stretched to the size of a hot air balloon.

When I finally came back, he turned to another machine with what looked like a long, thin willy and put a condom over it.

'If you can bend your knees, put the soles of you feet together and drop your legs to the sides like a frog. It won't hurt.'

Then he advanced on me with it. Visions of painful smear tests sprang to mind. OK, it looked thin and pretty harmless, but they always said having a speculum inserted didn't hurt and it bloody well did.

I took a deep breath and closed my eyes. Then fufu cam was in and I opened one eye, trying to look at the screen again.

After a few minutes, he said, 'Good. I can't see any problems. The only cause for concern at the moment is your ovulation, but I'll know more when I do the HSG test to check for any blockages or scarring on your fallopian tubes. If you'd like to get dressed again, the nurse will take you into the treatment room and get you set up.'

The nurse put the pictures he'd taken in a cardboard folder and handed them to me before leading the way.

OK, one test down, one to go.

'Did you take some Ibuprofen before you came as instructed, as the test can cause mild cramping?' she asked.

'Yep.' In fact, I'd taken four, just to be on the safe side.

Please let it be OK, Zelda.

I lay down on the second couch of the day in a bright white room with my legs up in stirrups.

'I'm just going to insert a speculum inside your vagina,' Dr Dye said, 'Then I'll wash your cervix with a special soap and insert a tube up into your uterus. Next, I'll put some X-ray dye through the tube to see if it flows freely, or if there are any blockages. OK?'

Did I look OK? I was going to have dye inserted up my fufu by Dr. Dye!

'Mmm,' I mumbled, wishing he would hurry up and get a move on.

I clenched my eyes shut as he inserted the speculum.

'Just relax,' he said.

Stop saying that! I opened my eyes and glared at him.

He peered into my cervix for a while with deep concentration.

'The tube is going in now,' he said. 'When I insert the dye you may get some cramping sensations.'

Hmmm, better not mention the dye to Karl in case he gets paranoid about getting a coloured willy when we next have sex and it puts him off.

'Dye going in now,' he said.

I hope he means the colour dye going in and not himself. Aghhhhhhhhhhhhhhhhhhhhhhhhhhhhhhhhhh!

It felt like a million razors had just shot up inside me. Mild cramps? Was he freaking joking?

I broke out in a cold sweat as he stood up and walked around to a booth. 'I'm just going to take some pictures now. I may ask you to move into another position. Just relax.'

Fuck off! How can I relax?

I squeezed my eyes shut and tried to block out the pain. Oooh, ah, oooooooooh. Not good.

Take your mind off it. Think about something else.

Chocolate. Nope, not working.

Jimmy Choos. Who cares? Ouch!

Fluffy kittens. My toes clenched in pain.

Punching the doctor. That worked slightly.

'Turn onto your right side,' Dr Dye said.

No. I don't want to move.

I bit my lip and turned over.

'Not long now,' he said.

Oh. My. God.

'And turn onto your back now.' He came out of the booth and sat down in front of me. 'Tube and speculum coming out now.'

About time!

'There. All done. That wasn't so bad, was it?'

If I hadn't had my legs strapped into stirrups, I would've kicked him in the head.

'Just lie here for about ten minutes and the nurse will bring you to my office to discuss everything.'

The nurse inserted a pad between my legs and removed them from the stirrups after the doctor had safely left the room. Hmmm, probably someone had kicked him in the head before and he was onto that number.

'You might get some spotting for a few days. That's perfectly normal,' she said.

I wasn't listening, though. I was too busy cramping.

Twenty minutes later, I sat in his office, staring at a model of the female reproductive tract and trying to ignore what felt like the period pain of an elephant.

'Now, I've looked at the X-rays and your tubes are all clear, so there's nothing to worry about there.' He put the X-rays to one side and examined another sheet of paper. 'This is your husband's sperm test results.' He handed it to me to look at.

Words like morphology, motility, and pH swam in front of my eyes.

He caught my worried look and gave me a reassuring smile. 'Everything is fine there, too. He has excellent sperm.' He leaned back in the chair and steepled his fingers. 'So, I'm going to prescribe Clomid for you to stimulate ovulation. I'll start you on the minimum dose of 50 mg, and you need to take it on days five to nine of your cycle.'

Why the minimum dose? I wondered, calculating the next date I could start it, which could be another three or four months, depending on my cycle. Four months! This was getting ridiculous. It was OK for him to sit there and dish out the tablets, but what about me? It had already been ten months and nothing. Nada. Zip. Zilch. He didn't understand the agonizing wait for something to happen. The high of hope that this could finally be the month, followed by the low of desperation and depression when your period arrived. He didn't understand the crazy and irrational, hormone-flying-around thoughts, that if you didn't get pregnant this month you'd just curl into a ball and die. My periods were all over the place, so my hormones were shot to bits. He didn't understand this unexplainable ache inside me to be a mother that literally consumed me at times. It was like my heart was being gnawed away. Yes, he was a gynaecologist, but he wasn't going through what I was going through. How could he? He was a man.

Part of me wanted to smack him over the head with his model fufu, and part of me wanted to burst into uncontrollable tears.

'Can't I just start at the higher dose and get on with it?' I pleaded as the waterworks began.

He shook his head. 'We have to start you on the lower dose. Increasing it can actually make conception more difficult.' He passed me a box of tissues from his desk as if it were the most normal thing in the world to have a thirty-three year old woman blubbing in his office.

I took one and sniffed loudly, cringing with embarrassment.

'You should ovulate five to nine days after the last tablet of Clomid. When you start taking the first dose, I want you to book another scan for day ten of your cycle and we can see if you're ovulating.' He started writing some notes down on a pad in front of him. Then glanced up and said, 'We

56

don't normally prescribe it for longer than six months.'

I gulped. 'Why?' Which came out more of a parrot-like squawk.

'One of the side effects is that, if you take it for longer than six months, it can make the lining of your uterus too thin, which will make it even more difficult to conceive.'

I slumped forward in the chair, deflated, struggling to cope with this new information. It was like giving you help with one hand but taking it away with the other.

'But don't worry about that now,' he said brightly.

Ha! Easy for him to say. The clock was ticking before I'd even started any actual fertility treatments.

'There are still other options you can try in the future: IVF, egg donation, surrogacy. Make sure you eat a healthy diet, get plenty of sleep. And remember, Gina, relax.'

I glanced at the model fufu one more time. If I aimed right, I could get him smack between the eyes.

Fuzzy Duck

Karl found me lying on the sofa, staring into space with unblinking eyes. The cramps had subsided to a dull ache but it still wasn't exactly what I'd call a pleasant way to spend an afternoon.

'I've been phoning all afternoon.' He stood over me, eyebrows furrowed together, concern plastered all over his face.

'I didn't feel like talking.'

He sat down next to me and pulled me into his arms. 'What happened?'

I filled him in on the latest.

'Well, that's good news, isn't it?' he said. 'At least they didn't find too much wrong, apart from the ovulation, and the drugs will fix that, right?'

I couldn't even bring myself to say what I was thinking: What if they didn't work?

'You just need to be more positive,' he said.

Yeah, yeah, my womb is a flower. Blah, blah, blah!

'I know!' His face lit up. 'Why don't we go away this weekend somewhere? Stay in a nice hotel and treat ourselves? A change of scene might get your mind off things.'

I perked up slightly at the thought of getting away from it all. It would be good to spend some quality time together instead of either getting snappy with each other because we were both under pressure, or me bursting into tears if an advert came on the TV for nappies.

But then I calculated my cycle. Dr Dye said I wasn't ovulating soon, so what was the point of going away and wasting a romantic weekend when the sex would be useless. No, it was better to save that for when there was at least a chance it would work.

'Let's do it another time.' I forced a smile.

'OK, well how about we go out this weekend with our friends and have some fun? Have a drink, have a laugh. It's been a long time since we did that. Moping around the house isn't going to help things.'

I sighed, nestling closer to him. 'But then I'll be tempted to drink, and I just don't want to do anything that's going to jeopardize my chances.'

He was silent for a while before finally saying, 'Don't you think that constantly being down about things is going to jeopardize your chances more? That's not good for you, either. One night out isn't going to hurt. In fact, I think it would help you. Go out, get pissed, and come back and have normal sex again.' He winked at me.

Normal sex? I'd forgotten what that was like. I thought back to the days just after we got married before we'd even contemplated trying for a baby. Fast and furious, slow and sensual, christening every room in the house with wild abandonment whenever the mood took us. Passion, excitement, and spontaneity was the name of the game. And then afterwards, we'd lie in each other's arms as the sweat glistened off our bodies, talking, or laughing, or listening to the sounds of each other breathing. It was fantastic! Now my legs were swinging in the air the second after he came, and we might as well have been couple of farm animals being forced to breed. We needed to do something to get that passion back.

I thought about his suggestion for a moment. Tempting. Very tempting. And maybe he was right. It had been ages since I'd felt like the old me. I was in danger of losing myself in all this frustration. Yep, what I needed was a good night out and a reality check.

I sat up. 'You're right. Maybe we can get Kerry to come if she's back. I haven't seen her for ages.' Kerry was an air stewardess who worked funny hours, and we hardly ever got to see her anymore. 'A good night out with the old crew.' I nodded firmly. 'I'll phone them now.'

'Kerry!' I squealed as she walked in the pub that Saturday night. 'God, it's been ages!' I gave her a hug and turned to the guy she was with. 'And you must be?' Kerry hadn't said she was bringing anyone with her. It had been six months since she'd broken up with her last boyfriend, and not a hint of anyone new on the scene, although I didn't have a clue why not. She was petite, with long blonde hair and huge blue eyes framed by luscious lashes.

'Mark.' He gave us all a beaming smile and shook my hand.

I ignored it and gave him a hug instead. 'Any friend of Kerry's is a friend of ours. Come and meet the rest of the gang.'

There were introductions all round as I sipped my first wine in months, savouring the flavour. I'd only had half a glass and felt slightly tipsy already. What was I going to be like by the end of the night? Oh, well, that was what I was here for – to have fun and let my hair down.

'So when did you two meet?' Amelia asked Kerry and Mark.

Mark glanced briefly at Kerry, obviously smitten. Decked out in designer jeans, a smart shirt, gelled hair and just the right amount of aftershave, he'd certainly made an effort to meet us all.

'At work,' they both said in unison, then turned to each other and laughed.

Oh, God, I hoped he wasn't an air hostess, ahem, I mean air host. Weren't most of them gay? No offence to gay people, but Kerry had what I'd call a rocky love life. She never seemed to find the right guy, and I didn't want another one to break her heart.

'I'm a pilot,' he said.

'Wow!' Amelia said. 'I thought pilots were all stuffy and

boring.'

That earned her a jab in the ribs from Dan.

But Mark just laughed. 'Actually, most of them are a bit up themselves. No, I fly cargo planes, not the big boys. We're a lot more down to earth.'

'Well, you're in for an interesting night.' Karl slapped Mark on the back. 'It's been ages since we all got out and had some fun, especially Gina.' He glanced at me with a grin. 'So...tonight we need to play some drinking games to cheer her up.'

I groaned. 'Oh, God, I'm on my way already. I'll be under the table in about five minutes, snoring.'

'No complaints!' Dan said. 'I'm liking the sound of this. What did you have in mind, mate?' he asked Karl.

'The name of the game tonight is "Monitors,"' Karl went on as we all grinned at each other, waiting for more. Drinking games had played a big part in our past, and Karl and Dan always went to great lengths to try and outdo each other with the funniest ones.

I giggled. 'What?'

'We've all got to be monitors of some kind,' Karl explained. 'Gina, you can be statue monitor, Amelia, you can be toilet monitor–'

'Ew, I don't like the sound of that.' Amelia scrunched her face up, but Karl put his hands up and carried on.

'It's not as bad as it sounds.' Karl chuckled. 'Mark, since you're the new boy here, I'll let you do the honours of being drinking monitor. Dan, you can be hair monitor. Kerry, you can be...' he tapped his lips, thinking, 'shoe monitor. And I'll be fuzzy duck monitor.'

We all burst out laughing, waiting for him to give us the rules.

'OK, throughout the night we all have to carry out our respective monitor roles. So, whenever Gina makes a pose like a statue, we all have to copy her for at least ten seconds without moving. Amelia, if anyone wants to go to the loo, they have to ask you, and you have complete discretion

61

whether you let them, and, of course, you have to tell them how much of their drink they have to down before they're allowed to go. Mark, you have to tell everyone what they're drinking the next round. And if you say, down in one, to any of us, we have to do the honours and down the drink we've got. Dan, whenever you say "hair," we all have to mess up our hair. Kerry, you're shoe monitor, so whenever you say, we all have to swap one shoe with each other.' He paused, waiting for the rules to sink in. 'And whoever the last person is to do the challenges has to take a big gulp of their drink.'

'Ha!' I said. 'How are the boys going to get in our high heels?'

Dan nearly choked on his pint of beer with laughter just thinking about it.

'And,' Karl carried on, 'since I'm fuzzy duck monitor, we'll be playing a tongue twister game, and anyone who gets it wrong has to take a gulp of their drink.' He paused. 'Got it?'

Nods and smiles all round.

'Great!' Karl rubbed his hands together.

I turned to Amelia and Kerry. 'So what have you two been up to this week?'

'Hair!' Dan cried out with enthusiasm, keen to get the game started. He grabbed some of Amelia's black bob to put over his own bald head, which was hilarious, and we all got our phones out to take pictures.

Everyone else followed suit, laughing. I gave myself an unflattering centre parting. Kerry pulled all of her long hair over her face. Amelia couldn't do much with her choppy bob since half of it was being used as a toupee for Dan. Mark, who seemed to be pretty game, gave himself a fringe, and Karl, well, his closely cropped hair wasn't moving much, so he licked his hand and pushed it back.

'Ooh, I need a drink.' I waggled my empty glass around, feeling the wine going to my head big time and enjoying the sensation. I glanced at Mark who was drinking monitor.

'OK, we're all having wine this round,' he said, and the boys bundled to the bar to get our drinks.

As soon as he'd left, Amelia and I huddled closer to Kerry. 'So, how's it going?' I nodded in Mark's direction.

'He's really sweet.' Her beaming smile matched his. 'We've known each other for a while through work, just as friends, but we only bump into each other occasionally. Then he asked me out last week. I'm sorry I haven't managed to call you guys in ages. We're short staffed and I've been pulling lots of long-haul flights.'

'He looks nice.' Amelia checked Mark out.

'He is.' Kerry nodded dreamily in his direction. 'He's really thoughtful and funny. And we just seemed to hit it off as soon as we met.'

'Here we go, girls.' The boys handed us our wine.

I put mine down on the table and pulled a ballerina statue pose, arms above my head in an arc, standing on tiptoes. 'Ballerina!'

Everyone just about managed it, apart from Dan who couldn't balance and had to keep holding onto the table for support.

We all ignored the amused stares of the Saturday night drinkers and carried on.

'Can we stop now?' Mark grinned at me as his legs wobbled.

'No!' I cried with laughter as I looked around our crazy group, who looked like the *Nut Cracker* on ecstasy. God, I'd missed having a laugh like this. 'Five more seconds. And Dan, you were last so you need to take a huge gulp of your drink!'

'I can tell this is going to be a cazy night!' Mark grinned when I finally let them stop.

'We haven't done much of this lately,' Karl said to him. 'Gina and I have been trying for a baby without any luck so we've been living like nuns. I finally convinced her to get out and have some fun, so we're making the most of it.' Karl sipped his pint. 'You ever thought about having kids?'

63

Mark shrugged. 'Not really. I guess eventually, if I meet the right person, but I can't say I've really thought about it much.'

'Get a cat, they're much less hassle,' Dan joked.

Amelia tutted at him.

'Good idea.' Mark nodded. 'And much less expensive.'

Karl looked at me over the top of his glass and smiled. 'Gina and I didn't really think about having kids before, either, and now I can't wait to be a dad.'

Dan slapped Karl on the back sympathetically. 'So what sort of cargo do you fly, Mark?' he changed the subject, trying to divert the attention away from babies, yet again, and back to more lively conversation.

'It can be anything from animals to post. The weirdest thing I've flown was a lion from London Zoo to an animal park in Scotland for mating.'

'Shoes!' Kerry shouted, kicking off one of her six-inch red stilettos in Mark's direction.'

'You'd better not stretch it.' I grinned at Karl who was trying to get on my black wedged heel. 'They're expensive.'

Dan was heaving with laughter as he tried to get on Amelia's platform heel.

I glanced down at our feet and doubled over, almost snorting wine out of my nose. The girls looked like Charlie Chaplin with one huge, chunky man's shoe, and the boys, well…they could only just about get their toes in the girls' shoes and were teetering in mid-air, holding onto the table for support.

'You guys are nuts.' Mark let out a big belly laugh, shaking his head.

I drained my second wine and put my hand up. 'Please, Miss, can I go to the toilet?' I said to Amelia.

'Nope.' She shook her head at me.

'But I'm going to wet myself.' I bobbed up and down.

'OK.' She grinned, 'But only if you go with Karl's Caterpillar boot on one foot and your wedge on the other.'

I narrowed my eyes at her in fake anger. 'Ooh, that's

nasty!'

'*And* you have to take a big gulp of wine.' She wagged her finger at me.

I took a swig and staggered off to the toilets, although I wasn't too sure if I was swaying so much because of the different shoe heights or too much alcohol, and I was too amused to care about the peculiar stares I got.

When I came back, there were shots of Sambuca all round.

Oh, God, this was going to be a crazy night.

'Tongue-twister!' Karl shouted out. 'The rules of fuzzy duck are quite simple. We all need to stand in a circle, so gather round.'

We shuffled into position, grinning.

'I'll start off by saying "fuzzy duck," then, going round clockwise, the next person has to repeat it. We carry on going round in the same direction until someone says, "does he," at which point we change direction and go anti-clockwise and say "ducky fuzz," until the next person changes it back to "fuzzy duck." Got it?' He smirked.

'I'm ready,' Mark said.

'Well, you can do the honours and start,' Karl said.

'Fuzzy duck.'

'Fuzzy duck,' Kerry said.

'Fuzzy duck,' I giggled.

'Does he?' Karl said, sending it back to me again.

'Fucky duzz,' I snorted and slapped a hand over my mouth.

'Ha! Get a drink of wine down you,' Amelia cried.

'Thash wash a fun night,' I slurred as we arrived back at our house five hours later. I tried to put the key in the lock, fumbling away, but it wouldn't go in. Then I dropped it on the step. 'Oops. Who changed the locksh?'

Karl crouched down, swaying in the dark on the front step to find them. 'You've got odd shoes on!' He cracked up with laughter, pointing at my right foot that had my wedgie on, and my left foot that somehow had Amelia's platform on.

I giggled. 'How did thash happen?'

'I want cheese on toast!' he shouted.

'Shhhhhhhhh.' I pressed my finger to my lips. 'Neighbours.' I nodded towards the dark street.

'I want cheese on toast,' he whispered, finding the key. 'Da da!' He jabbed it into the lock and we managed to get it open.

'Good...ideeeeaaaaa.' I stumbled into the house and bumped into the back of him, which suddenly seemed the most hilarious thing in the world.

'Cheese on toast and normal sex. Perfect.' He pulled me up the stairs. 'No, let's start with the sex, then cheese on toast.'

'Jush let me go for a wee,' I slurred as Karl flopped on his back on the bed.

When I came back, he was fast asleep. I stared down at him, ran my fingers along his jaw, and smiled at my gorgeous husband. Then I pulled off my dress and zonked out next to him.

The Other Woman

Whenever I didn't want my period to arrive, it always reared its ugly head, and when I wanted it to arrive so I could start my Clomid, it seemed to take forever. In reality, it was three months after I'd had my tests. The day of our wedding anniversary to be precise. Even though it had been over a year since we'd started trying, I took that as a good sign from Zelda.

This was definitely going to work. Oh, yes, bring it on!

My womb is a flower! A pretty, spring flower!

As instructed, I popped my pills on days five through to nine, and had a scan booked for day ten of my cycle.

Dr Dye arrived as I was lying on the couch.

'Right, let's have a little look and see if you're ovulating.' He smiled down at me as the scan machine beeped to life.

He spent the next five minutes moving the fufu cam around in silence.

Please say I'm ovulating. Please say I've got hundreds of follicles just waiting to burst open and be inseminated. Come on, what are you waiting for?

'Good news.' He finally looked up at me. 'You have a couple of good sized follicles. You're likely to ovulate in the next three to four days.'

Hallelujah! Woo hoo! Hurrah! I could've kissed him. Instead, I skipped (yes, I actually skipped) out to the car park with a permanent grin stretched from ear to ear, saying hello to everyone as if they were my best friend. I ignored their has-she-just-been-let-out-of-the-mental-wing? looks. I didn't care. Finally, this was the month I was going to get pregnant. I knew it. I just had this unexplainable feeling it would happen. Well, that, and Zelda must be on my side now!

Yeeeee ha!

'So we need to have sex on Friday and again on Sunday,' I told Karl with a huge smile when he got home from work. It was amazing my mouth hadn't actually fallen off yet from so much smiling.

'Great!' He pulled me into his arms, jumping up and down. Then he stopped abruptly. 'Oh, shit.' His wide grin suddenly dropped off his face.

'What?'

'I've got that work team building weekend in Hampshire.' His sudden horror mirrored my own.

'OK, so just cancel it.'

'I can't cancel it. It's been planned for six months.' He slumped down on the chair at the kitchen table, running a hand through his hair. 'And I'm the boss. It's not like I can miss it. We're staying at the hotel in Hampshire on Thursday night, then driving back to work early on Monday morning.'

'No!' I cried. 'We have to do it this weekend.' I flapped my arms around, panic suddenly twisting in my stomach. 'Why don't I just come with you?' I suggested.

'You can't. No spouses are allowed. If you come, they'll all want their partners to come, and it's strictly a work thing. That's the whole purpose of team building. Get to know your fellow workers, and all that. And anyway, our company is trying to expand internationally at the moment and Adam Sandler will be flying over from America on Friday night to meet us all.'

'The actor?'

'No, not the actor. This Adam Sandler is a huge potential client that we're hoping to win. If we can break into the American market, it's going to be a fantastic opportunity. Apparently, the Americans love all that team building stuff. I'm sure Adam and his colleagues won't be too impressed if we're all distracted with our wives.'

'OK, so…' I paced up and down, trying to come up with a

68

solution. 'I'll just drive down to Hampshire on Friday, we can have sex in between your meetings and team building games, then I'll come back and drive down again Sunday. How's that?' It wasn't exactly a romantic weekend or anything, but then, sex was purely functional at the moment, so did it matter? A brief thought flitted into my head of my son or daughter asking where they were conceived. "Oh, it was a quickie, functional afternoon in Hampshire, darling." I shook the thought away. No, we had to do whatever it took.

He tilted his head, thinking about it. 'That could work.'

I clapped my hands together. 'Fab!' There was no way, absolutely no sodding way I was going to miss trying the first month I was actually ovulating. I only had five months of tablets left.

Karl had consulted his itinerary in great detail before we arranged when I should drive up:

Friday
10.00 a.m – Team building games: Balloon Activities, Helium Stick, Rope Knot Game (whatever they were – sounded a bit kinky to me)

12.30 p.m – Lunch

2.00 p.m. – Raft Building Exercise and Tug of War (yawn)

4.30 p.m. – Free time

6.00 p.m. – Pre-dinner drinks and meeting with Adam Sandler (yep, I knew it! It was just an excuse for a piss-up)

7.00 p.m. – Dinner

8.30 p.m. – Keypunch Game (I seriously hoped they weren't going to get drunk and punch each other's lights out)

There was a nookie window of opportunity between 4.30 and 6. Perfect. It would take probably an hour to drive there, but there was no way I was going to have a repeat of the seventy mile an hour sperm, so I left early, allowing plenty of time.

The hotel was spectacular – a real country retreat. Rolling

69

expanse of manicured gardens, wood panelling everywhere inside. Even the heads of several stags dotted around, which was a bit yucky. I could feel their eyes staring at me as I trotted through reception and took the lift to the fifth floor with my head down. If his colleagues saw me here, they might be a tad pissed off that I'd managed to tag along and none of their wives had. Mind you, I'd only ever met one of the guys he worked with, and I'd never met his boss, so it wasn't like anyone would really recognize me, but for some reason I was feeling nervous. Kind of like I was the other woman, and I was meeting Karl for a secret tryst. It was actually quite exciting for a change. Hmm...maybe we should do a bit of role-playing to spice things up a bit. OK, so we *had* to do it, which was getting slightly repetitive and boring. Especially since the no oral sex rule applied, and the best positions to allow the sperm better access to my cervix were limited. But why not take the pressure off *having* to perform by acting out? Good job I'd put on some sexy knickers for once. This particular pair of red and black lacy ones, which were little more than a piece of dental floss, really, hadn't seen the light of day since our honeymoon. Yes, this could be quite exciting.

I got out of the lift and walked down the thick-carpeted hallway to his room. I looked down at what I was wearing – short black skirt, knee-high boots, tight V-neck jumper with no bra for added arousal.

I knocked on the door. 'Room service,' I said in a husky voice.

I heard a movement from inside. 'Er...can you come back later, please,' Karl's voice said.

I frowned at the door. Then banged again, slightly harder. 'Room service,' I said, more insistent this time.

'Gina? Is that you?'

'No, it's your other woman. The one you're having a secret affair with.' I grinned to myself.

The door clicked open slightly and his eyeball poked out around it. He visibly relaxed. 'God, I thought it was the maid trying to seduce me.' He quickly looked up and down the hallway to make sure no one was watching and pulled me gently inside.

I shut the door, thrusting out my almost D cups. 'No, I'm not the maid. I'm…' I tried to come up with a sexy name, 'Verotica.' I raised an eyebrow and licked my lips suggestively.

'Huh?' He stood there, looking at me like I was talking Russian.

For God's sake. Did I have to spell it out?

'Verotica,' I repeated, nice and slow and sexy. 'Your other woman.' I winked at him.

'Ah, yes! Verotica, you naughty minx.' The penny dropped. 'Oh yeah, you're much better in bed than my wife.'

'Oi, don't push it!' I laughed back, glancing around.

There was a small sitting area with plush gold couches in the middle of the room. To the right of me was a full-length wall mirror, and directly opposite it, to the left, was an archway that led to the bed. And what a bed! A six-foot, four-poster bed with intricate wooden carvings and plump burgundy and gold cushions.

'Nice bed,' I said.

'I know.' He pointed at the mirror. 'And we'll be able to see ourselves having sex.' His eyes lit up. 'Kinky!' He took my hand and pulled me through the archway and onto the bed, laughing.

I pushed him onto his back, straddling him. 'So, Karl, what can I do for you that your wife can't?' I licked my lips, eyeing his crotch.

'Everything,' his voice dropped to a husky whisper as he ran his hands up my thighs.

'Well, I'm sure your wife does *some* things right.' I insisted, pulling my jumper over my head to reveal the lack-of-bra status.

'Yeah, but not like you, Verotica. You're hot!' With one quick move, he'd flipped me over onto my back and was kissing me everywhere. My lips, neck, ooh, that sexy spot

71

just above my collarbone that made me shiver.

And the next minute, all our clothes were on the floor in a tangled heap, and I was on top of him again. I tried to think of other thoughts to put me off coming until after he did so my orgasm would aid his Olympic swimmers on their journey.

What shall I cook for dinner tonight?

Oh, God, that's good. Mmmm, yes.

Should I buy those black boots I saw last week? Nah, I don't need another pair.

Damn, that is soooo nice.

Shall I stop off on the way home and rent a DVD?

Omigod, I'm going to…

I rolled over so I was on my back again. All the better for aiding and abetting sperm travel, you know.

Don't come yet! Noooooooooo. Stag's heads!

That put me off for a nanosecond.

I tried to imagine I was shagging Gordon Brown instead. That definitely did the trick! And my orgasm disappeared long enough for him to ejaculate inside me.

I opened my eyes and looked up at Karl who was staring down at me with a lopsided, sexy grin, and then my orgasm exploded.

Satisfied and sweaty, I grinned back, and then suddenly I heard a knock and the sound of the door opening.

Before I could cover up my almost Ds, not to mention other bits, I saw a balding man with glasses appear in the sitting area through the reflection in the mirror, closely followed by an older man.

'Karl, are you here? I'd like you to meet Adam Sandler,' the bald man said.

'Aghhhhh!' I cried, grabbing the sheet and covering up my modesty in case they happened to look through the archway into the bedroom. In my haste, I accidentally kneed Karl in the nuts and he let out a howl of pain.

'Hang on! I'll be out in a minute, Clive,' Karl's high-pitched voice said, which came out a cross between a mouse sucking helium and a cry of the banshees, as he fumbled around for part of the sheet that I wasn't using to cover up, too.

'Oh!' Adam gasped when he noticed our reflection in the mirror for the first time, and his brain registered what his eyes were seeing, closely followed by Clive's jaw dropping as he noticed, too.

'Clive, I…I…wasn't…expecting you at this time!' Karl struggled for breath through the pain.

Shit. Clive's his boss.

I cringed and pulled the sheet over my head as a hot flush of embarrassment seared through me, not that they could see that, of course, but I was pretty sure they'd seen plenty already.

'We had a meeting booked for me to introduce you to Adam before dinner,' Clive said, his voice turning from surprised to incredulous.

'I thought the meeting was…ouch…booked for six not…ouch…four-thirty!' Karl said.

'Well, Adam's flight got in early so I thought we'd stop by now. I did knock but the door wasn't shut properly so it just swung open.' Clive again. 'I wasn't expecting you to be otherwise engaged!'

Damn, in the excitement of role-playing neither of us had checked the door.

'This company was started by my family, and I still believe in traditional family values!' Clive's voice took on a deadly tone. 'Not only is this a company weekend that you're being paid for, but I'm sure that your wife would not be very happy about you carrying on with other women behind her back!'

And before Karl could explain further, I heard Clive muttering his apologies to Adam and the door slammed behind them.

Oops!

'Omigod.' I pulled the sheet down when they'd left, staring at Karl open-mouthed. 'Go and talk to him. Quick!' I

73

did ushering hand movements as Karl cupped his nuts and rolled back on the bed with his eyes clamped shut and his mouth open with no sound coming out.

'You've broken my balls,' he squeaked breathlessly.

'No! Ball-breaking is not an option! They have to be in top working order. What can I do? How about a bollock massage? A splint? I've got a nail file in my bag.' I dived off the bed to rummage through my bag.

'You've done quite enough already for one day.'

'It wasn't my fault!'

'You didn't shut the door properly!'

'Neither did you!' I said.

'That's because you enticed me with Verotica.'

'You have to talk to him now. What if you get fired? What if you can't get another job? The recession's looming its ugly head. No one's taking on new staff lately. We might lose the house because we can't afford the mortgage, and then what would we do? How could we afford a baby, then? What if we need to have IVF? How could we pay for it?'

Karl opened his eyes and glared at me. 'I'll talk to him in a minute, when the throbbing has subsided.'

Half an hour later, he scrabbled around on the floor for his clothes.

I got dressed and bit my nails as I waited another half hour for Karl to come back.

As soon as the door opened, I sprang off the bed like a Jack-in-the-box. 'What happened?'

Karl shut the door, eyes downcast, staring at the floor with a grave expression. 'He actually thought you were my bit on the side, which he wasn't impressed about. As you heard, Clive's got very strong old fashioned family values.'

'I hope you put him straight. What did he say about your job? Is it safe? Oh, bugger, what are we going to do? '

Then he threw his head back and roared with laughter. 'Of course my job's safe! When I explained we were trying for a baby, they were absolutely fine about it all. They told me to apologize to you for walking straight in like that. If they'd known you were there, they wouldn't have come in.'

I clutched my chest with relief.

'Actually, they both thought you had an incredibly hot body.' He raised an eyebrow.

I gulped. 'You're joking?'

He threw his head back and roared with laughter. 'Of course I'm joking!'

Friends and the Green-Eyed Monster

Fourteen days after the hotel saga I was pregnant! I knew it. I was definitely pregnant. My boobs were sore, I felt slightly nauseous at the thought of chocolate (not that I was actually eating any since Julia's diet, but a girl can dream, can't she?), and I was getting cravings for cauliflower (I mean, seriously, anyone who has cravings for cauliflower *must* be pregnant. It stands to reason).

Gone were the days when I bought single pregnancy test kits. Oh, no, now I bought them in bumper packs of five so I always had a hefty supply of them. I was addicted to them, although I hid my addiction by buying them from different chemists and supermarkets all the time so I didn't get sectioned by the infertility police.

Karl was cleaning his teeth in the bathroom as I peed on the stick, which was slightly difficult due to my shaky hands, although I'd perfected a wonderful midstream flow in all these months.

Placing the plastic wand on the side of the bath, we both hovered over it, not daring to breathe.

I closed my eyes.

My womb is a flower. My womb is a flower. Come on Zelda, give me two little lines on the stick. That's not too much to ask for, is it? I'll be a really good person forever. I'll give money to charity. I'll volunteer for community work. I'll work part-time in the Oxfam shop. Anything!

I couldn't bring myself to open them again. 'Tell me what it says,' I said to Karl with my eyelids squeezed together like they'd been Superglued.

I heard a deep sigh. 'It's negative.'

'What! No!' That got my eyelids flying open pretty quick. 'It can't be.' I picked it up and stared at it.

Yep, Karl was right. Negative. Not even a hint of two lines.

'Fuck!' I slumped onto the edge of the bath, head in my hands, tugging at my roots. 'But I feel pregnant. I must be. I know I…' my voice trailed off. Should I do another one just to make sure?

'It's probably the hormone tablets giving you those symptoms.' Karl sat down next to me, stroking my hair. 'Don't worry, babe. It's only the first month on the Clomid.'

One month down, five to go. Tick tock, tick tock.

I was so numb I couldn't even cry at first. Maybe I was in shock. I'd been so positive this was the month. I felt this hole in my heart getting bigger and bigger, engulfing me in the process.

I had to do a French manicure on Stella later that morning, and she told me that her sister had done IVF eight times and then finally got pregnant naturally. Eight times! Aagh! I couldn't stop the uncontrollable tears, then. Real shoulder-shaking sobs, complete with blocked up nose and laboured breathing. How embarrassing, crying in front of a client. She was really good about it, even though I smudged her nail varnish a bit.

When Kerry appeared on my doorstep at five o'clock I looked a mess. Red-rimmed eyes, blotchy skin, big fat nose that Rudolph would've been proud of.

'Hey!' I forced a smile as I swung open the door to let her in.

'God, are you OK?' Kerry's forehead wrinkled with concern. 'Have you got a cold?'

I sniffed. 'Yeah, I think so,' I fibbed. I wasn't in the mood for talking about it, and I was desperately conscious that I harped on about body temperatures, cervical mucus, periods, and a whole host of pregnancy related issues all the time, and nobody likes a grumpy, feel-sorry-for-themselves friend.

If I were Kerry or Amelia, would I want to be friends with me anymore? I was turning into an unsociable, self-obsessed person who could only focus on babies, or the lack of them.

'Oh, I'd better not give you a hug, then,' Kerry said. 'Don't want to catch it.' She followed me into the kitchen.

'Sorry, I haven't got coffee, but you can have peppermint tea, green tea, or some vile nettle tea that tastes like boiled underpants,' I said.

'Are they used or unused underpants?' She grinned.

'Used.' I held my nose and wafted a hand underneath it for emphasis.

'In that case, I'll have peppermint. I'm off the coffee anyway at the moment,' she said quietly.

'So how's Mark?' I put my happy face on and forced myself to smile. It was horrible of me, but at that moment, I really couldn't give a shit how Mark was. I'd just felt the familiar twingy cramps of my period arriving.

Fuckyshittybollocks!

'That's what I wanted to talk to you about.' She traced a circle on the kitchen table with her fingertip, not looking at me.

'Oh, wow, you're getting engaged?' I pulled out mugs, stuffed in a couple of teabags and poured over the boiling water.

'Er…not exactly.'

I glanced up at her odd tone of voice, which was a mixture of sadness and trepidation, and I knew what she was going to tell me.

I felt all blood drain from my face and pool in the tips of my toes. 'You're pregnant?'

She swallowed slowly and nodded, watching my face carefully to gauge my reaction.

For a few seconds I just blinked at her, hoping I was wrong. Or maybe this was all a horrible dream. Yes, that was it. In a minute I'd wake up and realize it was just my subconscious being a nasty git. How could that be fair? Kerry was a single career-girl. She didn't even want kids.

How could she get pregnant and I couldn't?

There was a fuzzy line between wanting to scratch her eyes out for having something that I wanted and being crushed by sadness. I wanted to be happy for her, but part of me hated her at that second. I felt the green-eyed monster of jealousy crushing me. Then I was consumed with incredible guilt. She was my friend, after all. I should be happy for her – supporting her in everything she went through in life. It wasn't her fault I was a useless excuse for a woman.

I took a long sniff, determined not to cry again, and plastered a huge smile on my face. Even if she didn't buy it, I was going to have a good go at seeming ecstatically pleased for her. 'Wow! That's great!' I said, which came out slightly more high pitched than anticipated. 'Really fantastic news.' I sat down opposite her, not quite holding her enquiring gaze.

She reached out and squeezed my hand in hers. 'I wanted to tell you myself, because I know with all the fertility treatment you're going through, it must be pretty difficult for you to hear it.' She let out a stiff laugh. 'Especially since I've never even thought of having kids before. I mean, this is a huge shock for me.'

'No, it's great news. Really.' I squeezed her hand back.

'Are you sure you're OK about it? You don't hate me?'

Yes, but it's not your fault. It's mine. I'm the failure. 'Of course not.' I blinked back the tears pricking my eyes. 'So how does Mark feel about it?'

She rolled her eyes to the ceiling. 'I haven't told him yet.'

'What? Why not?'

She withdrew her hand and cupped the steaming mug of tea. 'We've only been together a few months. This isn't exactly what I'd planned on. It's…well, a bloody shock, to be honest. A condom split on us one night, which must've been when it happened. I can't believe it's happened.' She exhaled a deep breath.

'But you two have been getting on great, haven't you?'

She nodded. 'Yeah, I think he could be the one, but it's

just so soon in our relationship. He's going to think I've done it on purpose to trap him or something. I don't know how to tell him. I keep going over and over the conversation in my head but nothing sounds right.' She rested her elbow on the table, rubbing her forehead. 'And you heard what he said in the pub that night. He's never even really thought about having kids, either. He would rather have a bloody cat!'

'I'm sure that was just a joke. I used to say stuff like that all the time before I was trying for a baby. I'm sure he won't think like that when he finds out.' I rubbed her arm, desperately hoping that was true. 'Well, how do you feel about it? Are you pleased?'

She shrugged. 'I think so. I've had a bit of time to get used to it. It's not like I can really think about anything else since I found out.' She let out a bitter laugh and paused for a sip of tea. 'I've never felt maternal before in the slightest, so it's not like I've ever seriously considered being a mum, either, but…well, somehow it just feels right. Although I'm not sure how Mark will react, and the thought of being a single parent scares the shit out of me.'

'It's not going to come to that, you'll see.' I squeezed her hand.

It was her turn to start crying, then, which set me off.

And as I hugged her tight, I actually started giggling at the irony of it all. Maybe I was slightly hysterical, I don't know, but here Kerry was by accident with a precious gift I could only dream about, and here I was. If that wasn't Zelda sticking two fingers up to me, then I didn't know what was.

'Look at the pair of us,' I said, giggling through my tears.

She started giggling then, too. 'Do you think it will work out OK? For both of us, I mean.'

'It has to,' I said with sudden determination, wiping away the tears. If Kerry could do it, so could I. So, fuck you, too, Zelda! I'm *not* going to be beaten.

'Do you think he'll leave me?'

I shook my head. 'I've seen the way he looks at you. He's

head over heels. But you have to tell him straight away.'

'I will.' She leapt up with determination. 'In fact, I'll go home and ring him now and ask him to come over so I can break the news.' She hugged me tight. 'Wish me luck.'

'Good luck,' I said, walking her towards the door. 'I'm sure it will be fine. You'll see.'

'He doesn't want to know me,' Kerry wailed down the phone early the next morning.

'Right. I'm coming over,' I said.

OK, so I was jealous as hell that she was pregnant but I had to take it like a woman and suck it up. She was my friend and she needed me. I'd thought of nothing else all night. I knew how difficult it would be to raise a child single-handedly. For a brief, insane moment, I'd even wondered if she would give it up for adoption, and maybe Karl and I could be its parents.

When I arrived at her apartment, Amelia was already there.

'She's in the lounge.' Amelia let me in with a sombre smile.

I found Kerry curled up on her sofa with balled up, soggy tissues all over the place.

'What happened?' I sat on one side of her, stroking her back, as Amelia sat on the other side and handed her the box of nearly empty tissues.

'After I left you yesterday, I asked him to come over,' Kerry said in between sniffs. 'I mean, there isn't really an easy way to put it, is there? It's not like you can pussyfoot around it by saying, "Which restaurant do you fancy going to tonight, and by the way, I'm pregnant." So I just came out and told him straight.'

I nodded sympathetically as she spoke.

'His face turned whiter than this tissue.' She held up the new one she'd just massacred. 'At first, he didn't say anything. I think he was probably in shock, too. And then he said he needed to think about things and he'd call me later,

81

but he hasn't, so he obviously doesn't want to know me or the baby.' Her shoulders shook as tears streamed down her face.

I hugged her to me as Amelia took on back rubbing duty.

'Maybe he just needs a bit of time. I'm sure he'll phone you,' I said, trying to make her feel better. What did I know? I didn't know Mark as well as she did. I just hoped for her sake it was true.

'I bet he thinks I did it on purpose,' Kerry said. 'But it was an accident.' She rubbed at her stomach, as if the little life inside could hear her. 'I never meant for this to happen, honestly.'

'Sssh,' I rocked her. 'Of course you didn't.'

'What are you going to do?' Amelia said gently. 'I mean, if things don't work out between you. Will you keep it?'

I took a deep breath while I waited for Kerry to speak. Was there a possibility she'd have an abortion? The thought chilled me inside. I respected every woman's right to choose, but it would just tear me apart if she got rid of it while I was trying so hard for a baby of my own. Would she give it up for adoption? And if so, could Karl and I take on responsibility? My mind started daydreaming about the possibility. Little Mia (the baby was a girl in my daydream) at her first birthday party. Karl and I had bought her a giant fluffy cat, and Mia's eyes lit up when she saw it. "Maaaaaaaaaaaa," Mia wailed, which was the first word she'd spoken, and I interpreted it in baby-speak to mean Mum. My eyes filled up with tears of happiness as I kissed little Mia on her chubby cheek and tickled her toes. Then Kerry's voice brought me tumbling back to reality, and I realized I had tears streaming down my cheeks.

'Yes. I know I've always lived for my job, and I always said I never wanted kids, but...this is my son or daughter we're talking about.' Kerry rubbed at her stomach and wiped her eyes on yet another tissue. 'Somehow it just feels right. I'm not getting rid of it.' She took a long sniff, straightening up her shoulders with determination. 'Even if I have to raise it on my own.'

I grabbed a handful of tissues from the box and wiped my eyes. Shares in Kleenex would be rocketing the amount we were using.

'I know it's going to be difficult, trying to raise it on my own, but if that's what I have to do, then...' Kerry gave us a grim smile. 'I'm just going to have to do it.'

'Even though you've only been with Mark a few months I've seen the way he looks at you,' Amelia said. 'He's smitten. I'm sure he just needs a bit of time to get his head around it and he'll be back.'

'What if I've messed everything up, though?' Kerry wailed again. 'I think he's the one. I've never met anyone I'm so compatible with. I feel like I know him better than any other guy I've ever met. And he's funny and sweet and kind. Knowing my luck, I've just gone and blown the one chance of happiness I've got with Mr Right.' She grabbed the last tissue in the box and blew into it loudly.

A knock at the front door interrupted her sniffing-fest. Kerry's eyes lit up. 'Maybe it's Mark!'

'I'll get it,' I gave her arm a reassuring squeeze and opened the door.

Mark stood on the doorstep looking like he hadn't slept for a month. His hair stuck out at all angles. Dark bags circled his eyes. In his hand, he held a huge bunch of flowers.

'Er...can I come in?' He stood nervously, shifting from one foot to the other.

'Of course.' I followed him into the lounge.

Kerry's eyes lit up when she saw him, but I could see she was nervous. 'Hi,' she said softly.

'Right, well we'll just get out of your hair.' I dragged Amelia out of the room and motioned for Kerry to call me later.

'What do you think?' Amelia said to me as we got into our cars. 'Do you think they'll work it out?'

'God, I hope so.'

Neurotic? What, me?

Before I got out of bed on day twelve of my cycle, I reached my hand out from beneath the duvet, fumbling for the white digital thermometer on my bedside table with sleepy eyes. I popped it in my mouth and performed my morning ritual, waiting a minute until it beeped at me with a reading. Then I recorded it on a chart by my bed and compared it with the previous days' results. No ovulation yet, which meant we would probably need to have sex today. Oh, what joy!

That afternoon I was in the bathroom and discovered the arrival of my egg white goo. Hey presto, it was here! I peed on the ovulation predictor kit, just to be sure. Yep, I was about to ovulate.

I phoned Karl at work to tell him. Since he was in some big important meeting or other, I left a message on his voicemail and clock-watched through the hours until he got home.

'What a bloody day!' Karl came home at 8 p.m. as I was pacing the floor. Eight o' clock! Didn't he know the urgency? I was ovulating for God's sake. What if we missed it? What if my follicle popped out and we hadn't even done it yet? It would be another month lost. It didn't bear thinking about.

'Where've you been?' I verbally pounced on him as soon as he got through the door.

'And hello to you, too. I've been at work.' He dumped his briefcase on the kitchen table and opened it, spreading out various bundles of paper. 'Clive's sprung a big presentation on me for tomorrow morning. I've got to get these reports done tonight.' He loosened his tie and sat down, bending his head over all the paperwork. 'Is dinner ready? I'm starving.'

'No, I thought we'd eat later. We need to have sex.' I stared at his hunched-over back as he grabbed a pen and scribbled furiously like he hadn't heard me. A few minutes passed before I said, 'Did you hear me?'

'Huh?' He didn't look up.

'We need to have sex. Now.'

'I've got reports to do. Let me just finish this and then we can have sex.' He shuffled bits of paper around.

'No, we need to have it now. What if I miss ovulating?'

'Later,' he said firmly. 'A few hours won't make that much difference.'

'Actually, it might. That's the whole point. There's no point in taking all these horrible drugs if we're not going to get to the sex part. We need to do it now!'

He swung around, his facial muscles hardening. 'For fuck's sake, Gina, a couple of hours isn't going to make a difference.'

'Yes, it might. Come on, it won't take long. We'll just have a quickie and you can get back to your reports.' My voice quavered with a sudden panic. We had to do it now. Now. Not later. Right this second. Premature follicle popping was not an option! Why didn't he understand the urgency? The timing was crucial.

'No. It won't make a difference.' He narrowed his eyes at me, his voice sharpening. 'When are you going to realize that the world doesn't revolve around you? People have got other things to do than have bloody sex whenever you say! This is a very important presentation. God, I'm under pressure from you, under pressure from Clive.' He turned his back on me and resumed scribbling. 'Do you remember when we actually used to have lives that didn't revolve around getting pregnant?'

I felt myself getting hotter and hotter, simmering away under the surface. It didn't matter what he thought. When we had a baby, all of this would be worth it. 'But we might miss ovulation. It's all right for you. You're not the one who has to take all these bloody tablets all the time that mess up your hormones. All you've got to do is turn up and ejaculate.' I tried to stay calm but heard my voice cranking up a couple of notches. 'I'd say you've got the easy end of the deal, wouldn't you?'

He threw his pen down on the table and stood up, turning to face me. 'No,' he yelled back. 'I wouldn't, since I have to put up with your mood swings and neurotic behaviour!'

'I'm not neurotic! One of us has to make sure we know when the right time is. I'm just being practical, not neurotic.' Yes, that was it. I was just using my common sense, so, in fact, I was actually being very level-headed about the whole thing. 'I'd love it if men were the ones who had to get pregnant. Ha! I'd like to see you have to check for egg white every month and deal with too much testosterone flying around all the time so you had sudden urges to strangle people. Or have acid dye blasted up the end of your willy after it's been gauged open by a speculum!' Then I bit my lip to avoid blurting out anything else in anger. I had to walk on eggshells around him so I didn't upset him in case he refused to have sex with me. God, that sounds terrible, doesn't it? He'd never actually refused to have sex with me when it was the right time of the month, but he hated all the sex-to-order. Hell, so did I! After all this time, it's like we're just going through the motions, like robots. And now it always seems like there's something hanging between us, whether it's stress, drugs, fear, resentment, I can feel it, and I know Karl can, too.

He started gathering all the papers up and stuffing them back in his briefcase.

Great, finally he was getting the message. Sex. 'Come on, then,' I said. 'Shall we go upstairs?'

He pressed the locks closed on his case with a loud click. 'No. I'm not going upstairs. I'm going somewhere that I can finish this work in peace. And the last thing I feel like doing right now is having sex with *you!*' He spat out the last word like I was some kind of leper. And before I could tie him down or rugby tackle him to the floor to have sex, he stormed out, slamming the front door.

I stared down the empty hallway. What was I going to do now? No, no, no. I couldn't miss out this month. We had to do it. Agh!

I picked up my mobile and texted "Sorry."

No reply.

I left it five minutes then texted "Really sorry."

Nothing.

I managed to wait another ten minutes then sent, "Really, really, really sorry.'

Deafening silence. I looked at my phone to make sure it had a signal or the battery hadn't died.

Nope. Everything was in working order.

Half an hour went by, then I texted. "Love you."

Ten minutes later, I still hadn't had a reply so I phoned his mobile. It rang and rang, then went to voicemail.

Bugger. I'd just have to leave a message. 'Look, I'm really sorry about that. It's just that it feels like time is running out, and it's not like I can accurately predict when I'm going to ovulate, so we need to make sure your sperm is already there when it does. Can you come back, please?'

Nothing.

Half an hour later, I sent him another text. "Please come back."

Nothing.

We didn't normally fight. I know that sounds weird, but it's true. Before all the hormones turned me into a paranoid Looney Tune, we hardly ever had a crossed word. All I wanted him to do was come back and hold me. Tell me everything would work out.

I rang again another ten times and they all went to voicemail. OK, so maybe that was the slightly neurotic behaviour Karl was talking about, but I was a woman on a mission and a woman obsessed. And that was the thing about obsession – it escalates and can't be controlled. You're absolutely and utterly powerless to do anything to stop it.

When it got to 11 p.m., I was flitting between worry and anger.

How dare he walk out on me when it was the right time of the month!

Oh, no, what if he's been in an accident!

This is so unfair of him to punish me. It's not like I'm asking for much – only his willy.

Where the hell is he? Is he OK?

Bastard.

I sat on the bottom step in the hallway, staring at the door, willing him to come back.

Please, Zelda, make him come back and have sex. I know you're probably getting pissed off with me, too. But...

My ears pricked up at the sound of his key in the lock.

As he opened the door, he stood there staring at me.

I stared back.

'I'm sorry,' we both gushed at once.

I rushed into his arms where he enveloped me in a warm hug.

'Where've you been?' I asked.

'Down the pub.'

'Did you finish your reports?'

'Yes.' His fingers stroked my back. 'Gina, you have to calm down. You're driving me crazy.' He shook his head sadly.

I nodded into his shoulder, unable to speak. I was driving myself crazy, too. At this rate, I'd be in the loony bin in a few months. 'I know.' I nuzzled into his neck, gently kissing the top of his ear. 'But it's a complete nightmare being pumped full of hormones. You don't know what it's like. It's like I've been taken over by the Invasion of the Body Snatchers. One minute I'm bawling my eyes out, and the next I want to murder perfectly innocent people. I've got no control over my emotions anymore. I know I've been a pain in the arse lately, but timing sex around ovulation is absolutely essential.'

'I know it's tough on you, and I know how desperately you want this, but unless you start to chill out a bit it's not going to get us anywhere.' He picked me up in his arms and carried me upstairs.

Chi and Rabbits

All these months everyone had been telling me to relax, which actually had the opposite effect on me. It made me want to murder them in very slow, painful ways.

But, deep down I knew they were right, which meant I needed to do something drastic to help before I ended up mad. Well, madder than I already was.

So when my period arrived yet-a-bloody-gain, I decided I needed to start taking action. And who better to call than Poppy?

'Can you recommend anything holistic that will increase my fertility and relax me?' I asked her over the phone.

'Oh, yes. There are a lot of things that might help. Feng Shui can increase fertility energy in your environment around the house. Acupuncture has achieved a high success rate with infertility. It's especially good to combat stress and rebalance yourself. Or you could try yoga for calmness and wellbeing. Honestly, I think this could be just what you need.'

'OK, great.' I scribbled everything down.

'It's up to you if you want to try one thing at a time or everything at once. It can't hurt.'

Hell, yeah. No point beating around the bush. I was going to do everything at once!

'Thanks, Poppy. Any news with you yet?'

'No,' she said, although her voice was as upbeat and positive as usual. 'It will happen when it's right. We're going to start another round of IVF soon.'

'Well, I've got my fingers crossed for you. I'll phone you soon.' I hung up and got straight on the Internet to look for a

Feng Shui practitioner near me.

At 3 p.m. the next day Amanda Groves, feng shui Consultant to the stars, no less, was on my doorstep. According to her website, she'd feng shuid top actors and actresses, as well a few models and singers, so she must be pretty good at her job.

She was younger than I thought. Probably the same age as me, with bright red curly hair that screamed of energy and abundance.

'Hi.' She extended her hand with a beaming smile and gave me a warm handshake.

'Hi. Come in.' I waved her in.

'Actually, before I start I have to point out something to you.' She turned around and looked over her shoulder behind the front entrance.

I followed her gaze. All I could see was a small silver birch tree, a wall, and then the street.

'In feng shui the front door is the mouth of chi, which means it's where all the energy enters your home. You should ensure there's nothing in direct line with the door, such as a tree or street or other object, that can block the flow of positive energy. It needs to be a clean and beautiful area.'

'Right.' I scratched my head. 'I could always cut the tree down.' But what about the street? Not much I could do about that, except move house.

She turned back to me and nodded. 'Yes, that would help a great deal.'

I took her jacket and hung it up as she looked around the hallway with critical eyes.

'Let's start downstairs and then finish in the bedroom, which is one of the most important areas for fertility,' she said.

I grabbed a pad and paper and followed her around.

'You should put a brass wind chime in the entry way to welcome energy into the house,' she said.

I scribbled that down furiously.

'And plant a fruit tree in the back garden, away from the door. Fruit trees are an ancient symbol of fertility, and the more fruit they bear, the higher your chances of conceiving.'

'OK.' Maybe I could cheat and buy one with loads of fruit on already.

'The whole idea of feng shui is to create a sense of inner harmony and balance in your life, promote positive energy, and protect you from negative forces,' Amanda said.

'Well, I definitely need a hefty dose of harmony.'

She wandered into the lounge and eyed a wilting peace lily in the corner. 'You need to make sure all plants in the house are well cared for.'

I grabbed a glass of water from the coffee table and poured it into the pot. Da da!

She frowned at some *Baby Expert* magazines and *How to Get Pregnant* books, haphazardly left open on the coffee table, and Karl's dirty socks on the floor that he'd left there the night before. 'You need to ensure the whole house is clutter-free. Clutter depletes the chi energy and may make it difficult to conceive,' she said.

I jotted that down: No stinky socks or books to be left out.

Eyeing the sofa in front of the window she said, 'Hmm.'

Oh, God, what did that mean? Would we have to buy a new sofa because the old one wasn't chi friendly?

She pointed at it. 'The windows should remain unblocked to allow the chi to flow without bumping into things. You'll need to move the sofa.'

I stared around the room. Right, so I could just move it to the opposite side of the wall. But then it would mean rewiring the TV and stereo that were in the way. Never mind, Karl could do that.

She pulled out a compass and studied it with thought, glancing up now and then. Next, she pointed to one side of the house. 'This is the west sector, which is associated with children. You need to put something in the west areas of the house like a bright light, candles, white flowers, and fresh fruit.'

Got ya!

An hour later, we ended up in the bedroom.

Out with the compass again. 'Your husband should sleep with his head facing the northwest, so you'll need to move the bed over there.' She pointed to one wall.

She knelt down and peered under the bed, then let out a small gasp.

Uh-oh. I didn't even want to think about what was under there. I hadn't cleared it out since we'd moved in five years ago. I usually just Hoovered around everything underneath it.

I knelt down next to her. An exercise mat, piles of books, a bicycle pump and a very uncomfortable looking bicycle seat (that was on Karl's side; what the hell was that doing there?), some dumbbells, a box of photos and mementoes from Mum, and a cheese grater (Oh, that's where I'd put it! I'd been looking for that for ages. These hormone tablets were making me forgetful, too).

'You have to move everything out from under the bed and keep it clear. Don't store anything under there at all.' She smiled at me. 'Normally, you need to make sure the house is completely clean and clear. No dishes left in the sink, windows cleaned inside and out regularly, sinks and toilets in good working order, everything clutter-free. But with this area we're going to break one of the feng shui rules.' She paused, making sure she had my full attention. 'Once you've cleaned it, don't touch the area again until after the baby is born.'

Well, obviously I wouldn't have any problem breaking that particular rule. And anyway, in my defence of being an undomestic goddess, I'd been far too busy lately trying to get pregnant to worry about cleaning. I mean, seriously, what was more important?

'If you sweep or Hoover under the bed once you activate the lucky fertility energy, you'll be undoing all the positive chi you've attracted.' She looked at me sternly to make sure that sank in.

I made a note of it just in case I suddenly developed a mad under-the-bed cleaning urge. Not likely, but then anything was possible with my hormone-infested brain lately.

'Pomegranates,' she said.

'Er…pardon?'

'Pomegranates are a symbol of fertility. If you get a picture with a pair of pomegranates on them, sliced open, that will bring you good luck.'

'Check,' I said, writing it down. God knows what Karl was going to think about that.

'Elephants, storks, and rabbits are also associated with fertility. You could get a pair of elephants and place them on either side of the bedroom door. Or a pair of rabbits.'

Well, I already had a pair of Rabbits in my bedside drawer. Rampant Rabbit Thrust Deluxes, no less. Surely I'd get double points for those.

'And put a pair of dragons on your husband's bedside table,' she said.

Half an hour later, she'd gone, and I was straight on the phone to Kerry and Amelia to see if they fancied a shopping trip on Saturday.

Karl arrived home at 7 p.m. after I'd had a frantic clear out and furniture rearranging session.

'What's happened to the tree?' He found me in the bedroom, hot and sweaty, pulling out the last of the stuff from under the bed.

'It was blocking the chi,' I said.

He just nodded at me slowly. 'Right. And why are your vibrators on either side of the bedroom door?'

'Rabbits are fertility symbols,' I said, as if he really should know better.

He looked at me like I'd just told him his head was on fire. 'God, I need a drink.'

WWF Wrestling

Kerry, Amelia, and I were in Starbucks in town on Saturday. I eyed Amelia's caramel latte, my mouth watering with lust. How long had it been since I'd had one? I couldn't even remember now. I stared down at my iced rooibos tea that tasted like gone-off urine. Not that I've ever tasted urine, you understand. Yes, I'd contemplated some weird things in my quest to get pregnant, but drinking urine definitely wasn't one of them. Even though I saw on the Internet there was this African tribe in a village in the middle of nowhere that swore by it. Apparently, they had the most fertile women in the whole country because of their wee-drinking fetish. Popping them out like there was no tomorrow, they were. No, I'd just stick to my feng shui shopping list for now.

Kerry looked a lot happier than I'd seen her the other day. Not a puffy eye or sniffy nose in sight.

'Well…?' I tilted my head, prompting Kerry to give us the latest.

She clapped her hands together and grinned like a loved-up teenager. Then she held out her left hand so we could inspect the huge rock on her ring finger. 'He proposed.'

'Bloody hell!' I said as Amelia and I stared at it with appreciation. 'Omigod! I'm so happy for you.'

'That's fantastic,' Amelia said. 'Come on, we want all the juicy gossip. What happened when we left?'

'He said it was a big shock for him. That he did want to settle down and have kids in the future, but this was a bit sudden, and it had taken him completely by surprise, which is why he had to think about it for a while.' She paused for breath. 'I mean that's understandable. But he said he knew I was the girl for him, even though we'd only been together for three months. Under normal circumstances he would've waited longer to propose, but now this has happened, he said what was the point in wasting any more time when he knew it was right, and...' She glanced down at her ring, a goofy smile plastered all over her face. 'He wanted to make a commitment to me and show how much he loved me, and that he was going to be there to support me.'

I stared at the happiness radiating from her face. OK, so it was sudden and unexpected, but who was to say it wouldn't work out between them? If they loved each other enough, and I suspected they did, that was all that mattered. I had a good feeling that everything would be fine, and I was genuinely happy for her. But, deep down, the green-eyed monster reared its ugly head. I stared at her still-small stomach and felt a knife of jealousy stab me in mine.

'When's the wedding?' Amelia asked. 'I hope we're both going to be bridesmaids. Then she pulled a face. 'As long as you don't make me wear a ginormous puffy dress that makes me look about twenty stone.' She grinned.

'You two are *definitely* going to be bridesmaids. And we thought we'd wait until after the baby is born to tie the knot. I don't really want to be pregnant in my wedding pictures, and I think we need a bit of time living together before we get married. He's moving the first of his stuff in tomorrow,' Kerry said.

'Wow, it's so exciting,' Amelia cried.

'Now I just have to tell my mum. She'll freak. She didn't even know I was seeing anyone, let alone that I'm pregnant and engaged.' Kerry grimaced at the thought.

'And how are you feeling?' I nodded at Kerry's stomach. 'Any morning sickness yet?'

'Nope. Nothing. I just feel full of energy. It's amazing. Now, enough about me.' She smiled at me. 'What's on your feng shui shopping list?' She squeezed my hand to let me know she knew how hard it must be to deal with all her pregnancy stuff.

I pulled my list out of my bag. 'A pair of elephants, a pair of dragons, a wind chime, two pictures of pomegranates, a fruit tree, and candles.'

Amelia downed the last of her latte. 'Aren't you drinking that?' She tilted her head towards my wee tea.

I scowled at it. 'It's yuck.'

'Come on, then, let's go and get your stuff.' Kerry stood up and gave me a hug.

Five department stores, one DIY store, and about a million other stores later, I only had one thing left to get: The pair of elephants. Everyone must've been on a wild elephant-buying spree lately because there were none anywhere.

'This is the last shop we can try.' Amelia stood outside a knick-knack shop at the far edge of town.

Inside, we browsed the Indian wood carvings, glass candle holders, and furniture, trying to ignore a gigantic woman (who could've been Hulk Hogan in drag, I wasn't entirely sure) shouting at her two kids.

'Pack that in, or I'll give you a smack round the head,' she said to a snotty-nosed boy of about six who had picked up a carving of a snake. 'You stupid little brat,' she said to a sweet-looking girl of about four, whose hair was matted and dirty.

'But I'm not doing anything, Mummy,' the girl said, then tried to hug her mother's legs.

Hulkess pushed the girl away. 'Get off! I'm getting bleeding sick of you both.'

Distressed, the girl stood in the shop and burst into tears, looking at her mum with longing.

'Can I have this?' the boy held up the snake to his mum.

'No. You're not getting anything. You got something for your birthday. You'll have to wait until Christmas to get more. And stop asking me for stuff all the time.' Hulkess roughly pulled the boy away from the snake and then promptly ignored him.

I glared at her.

The little girl's sobs were getting louder. 'Can I have a cuddle, Mummy?' She looked up at her mum with huge, dark eyes that were so sad they made me want to scoop her up and run off with her.

Hulkess didn't even look up from examining the tea light holder she had in her giant hands. 'No. You can have a smack if you carry on. Stop your sodding whinging, the pair of you. I've had enough.'

I quickly scoured the shelves, wanting to get out of there before I did something I'd regret, like smack the horrible woman over the head with a heavy wooden lion. How could she be so nasty to her children? And why was it some people who weren't fit to be parents, and didn't seem to care about their children, managed to be lucky enough to conceive? It just wasn't fair.

I was just about to give up hope of ever finding any elephants when I spied a plastic box that held two beautifully carved wooden ones.

As I reached out and grabbed the box with excitement, I saw someone else's hand appear in my line of vision and grab it at the same time.

I glanced up and saw Hulkess's fat sausage fingers holding onto the box.

'Er…excuse me, but I saw them first,' I said, tightening my own grip on the box. There was no way I was letting these babies go.

'No you didn't,' she said in a gruff voice.

'Yes, I did.' I pulled it towards me, but she didn't let go.

'Nah. I did.' She pulled it back towards her, almost popping my arm out of its socket.

'Give it back,' I said.

'No.' She glared at me. 'You gonna make me?'

'Mummy,' the little girl wailed. 'I need to go to toilet.'

'Shut up!' she snapped at her daughter without looking around.

'These are my elephants.' I pulled them back towards me

and narrowed my eyes at her, hoping there wouldn't be a full-on elephant fight. Hulkess would probably get me in a headlock or do a big body drop on me and I'd be a goner. But I was knackered from shopping, pissed off that everyone else in the world seemed to be able to get pregnant except me, and my hormones were going through the roof. Plus, the woman seemed like a complete bitch who didn't give a shit about her kids, and clearly wasn't fit to be a parent. I needed a fertility elephant more than she did.

'Oh, yeah? And who says so?' She stepped closer, her face menacingly close to mine as her top lip curled up.

I stuck my chin up in the air and straightened my back, hoping to appear taller than my five foot five. It didn't do much good, since she was still towering over me. Out of the corner of my eye, I saw Kerry, Amelia, and the tiny Asian woman who was serving at the counter, staring at me open-mouthed.

'I say so,' I insisted, my voice getting louder as I wondered what I could do to get them off her. Elbow her in the ribs? No, she probably wouldn't even feel it with all the meat on her.

'Mummy,' the little girl wailed. 'I need to go wee wee.'

'Shut up, you little bugger,' Hulkess snapped.

That just did it for me. I saw red, and a whole lot of other colours, too. I stamped on her fat foot as hard as I could with my high-heeled boots, grinding my heel in. Yes, I know, I know. That was a really horrible thing to do, especially in front of her poor children, but she deserved it.

She let out a scream and let go of the elephants, bending down to rub her foot. 'You fuckin' bitch.'

'Don't swear in front of your kids,' I hissed. 'You don't know how lucky you are to have them!' I stamped on her other foot just for using the F-word in front of them.

Before she could punch me in the face, or do a Hulk Hogan special on me, I ran past the Asian woman, threw twenty pounds on the counter, and legged it out of there.

Will I Ever Get Pregnant?

Another two periods later, I'd given up hope of the feng shui working. Karl didn't actually come out and say, "It was a ridiculous idea, and I told you so," but I knew that's what he was thinking. And it was pretty stupid. I mean, how could planting a fruit tree or buying a ridiculous pomegranate picture get you pregnant?

Poppy was regularly going on about *Spirit and Destiny* magazine that she bought, which had lots of horoscopes and feel-good articles about holistic health. Apparently, it had inspirational stories each month that covered guardian angels, mind and body well-being, white magic, spiritual healing, and experts in psychic phenomena. I did wonder, if it was written by psychics, then why couldn't they just telepathically send it to you, instead of printing up a whole magazine each month, but I was desperate, and maybe something in there would help me find answers about myself that could help. Was I really self-sabotaging? Was my fufu chakra blocked? Could I find a guardian angel to help me conceive?

After reading "How to unlock your intuition", "Open your spiritual cash converter", "Guardian Angels are all around you", "Natural ways to win the cold war", and "The new moon and you", I was none the wiser. I did, however, find some pages at the back with numbers for psychic hotlines that promised "Genuine psychic readings by proven and gifted mediums, psychics, and Tarot card readers." Yes, it was probably equally ridiculous but desperate times call for desperate measures.

"Will I get pregnant?" I quickly fired off a text to

ANGEL111.

I tapped my foot, waiting for a reply, wondering if I'd completely lost it this time.

"My magic ball of 6 says YES!" came the reply.

"Will I have more than one?" I fired back.

"My divination rod is aquiver with YES!" the text said.

"When?" I asked.

"The answer is YES! But keep it a big secret!" it read.

I glared at the phone. OK, maybe it was just a technical hitch. Maybe the mobile phone signals messed up their psychic vibes or something.

I tried another number.

"Will I get pregnant?" I rattled off.

"You will achieve your dreams," was the reply.

"When?"

"When the full moon is in the sky."

Which bloody full moon?

"Which month and year?" I texted, sighing with impatience.

"Yes."

Aghhhhhhhhhhhhhh!

I should've given up then, but I needed to get an answer. I turned to the text Tarot card reading numbers next. All I had to do was concentrate on my question, then text them, and I'd receive three tarot cards with the answer.

Five minutes later, I got a bunch of pinging text messages back.

The first one said: "Seven of Swords – Plans may fail. Success will not be complete."

The second one said: "The Chariot – Victory and success in your world."

The third one said: "The Knight of Cups – Look for a message or sign."

What did they mean? Would I fail or succeed? And why did I have to look for a message? That's why I was bloody texting them!

I clenched my eyes shut, concentrating on my question,

then texted another tarot line, waiting with bated breath for the reply.

"The Two of Swords: Relationships are rife with tension."

"The Ten of Cups reversed: Betrayal and failure. The loss of love and friendships."

"The Ace of Swords reversed: Loss and infertility are likely."

NO! No, no, no! I didn't like the sound of that one at all.

Maybe if I just tried another one…

Ooh, what's that? My eye caught a website in the back of the magazine that advertised spells. I quickly went online and looked up a fertility spell. What did I have to lose? I just wouldn't mention it to Karl, who thought my behaviour lately was bordering on insane.

I jotted everything down that I'd need:

A white candle
A green candle
Frankincense incense
A drawstring pouch
A rose quartz crystal
Sprig of fresh rosemary
A fresh egg
A fresh fig
A glass bowl
A sharp knife
A pen
A shovel
A symbol of your desire to have a baby (baby clothes, rattle, etc)

It was dark outside by the time I'd had a trip to the supermarket, New Age shop, and the shed. Finally, I was good to go.

I decided to do it in the bedroom, since that seemed more like a good place to magically enhance my fertility. After lugging everything upstairs, I read the instructions through carefully five times before beginning.

I sat cross-legged on the floor, placed the candles in front of me with a gap in the middle, and lit them. Then I worried that maybe I shouldn't have the bedroom light on in case the electricity interfered with the magic energy so I leapt up to turn it off, which then made it a bit difficult to see the instructions I'd written down.

OK, what next?

Put the egg on the left of you, the fig on the right, and the bowl in the middle. Then place the symbol of your desire to have a baby in front of the bowl.

Since I couldn't decide on only one appropriate symbol for my baby, I'd bought several: a gorgeous, soft pink teddy bear, two pairs of teensy pink socks, a pink dummy, and the cutest little pink baby booties ever. OK, so if it was a boy, it might have a few gender issues with all the pink going on, but I couldn't resist them.

I arranged everything carefully and looked at the next instructions.

Put a rose quartz crystal and some fresh rosemary in the drawstring bag and place it in front of the bowl.

Check.

Draw a fertility symbol or a symbol of your child on the egg.

Damn. What should I draw? It could be crucial to the whole thing. A dummy? A pram? What was the symbol of fertility? Was it one of those weird circles with a plus sign in it, or was I getting mixed up with something else? Should I draw a pregnant woman?

I tapped my lips with the pen. A willy! That was it. Didn't all those fertility gods have humongous willies? Yes, I distinctly remembered going to Dorset one summer with Karl and finding that chalk fertility symbol of a naked man on the hillside. His was huge!

I drew a big willy on the side of the egg, then sat back and studied it. Was that a clear enough message? Just in case the spell got lost in translation and gave Karl a penis extension or genital warts instead, I drew a baby. Because drawing had never been my strong point it ended up looking more like a cross between a kid with a square head and an elephant.

Break the egg into the bowl and place the empty shell on the left.

I made sure I didn't spill a drop down the side of it as I cracked the egg.

Make a small cut in the fig and carefully scrape the seeds into the bowl.

Hmm…this bit was a little messy. Fig juice ran down my hands and plopped onto the white carpet.

Crap! I rubbed at it with my finger, turning it into a blobby mess. I didn't want to stop the spell and get a cloth. If I interrupted it, who knows what might happen? I'd probably end up ruining it completely and being granted a lifetime supply of dishcloths by the magic kitchen fairy. I ignored the stain and carried on. I'd just move a plant pot over it if it didn't come out and hope Karl never noticed.

Place the rest of the fig into the egg shell. This represents the presence of your baby in the womb. Then put it on your left side.

I gouged out the flesh from the fig and patted it into the shell, being careful not to break the delicate egg.

With your finger, stir the contents of the bowl three times clockwise.

Did it matter which finger?

I used the gouging finger since that one was already dirty.

Repeat these words:

With this spell I call upon all good powers!

I call to the Goddess of life and ask you to hear me.

May the Goddess bless me with a child.

I bring love to start my family,

I bring energy to start my family.

Accept my small token of fertility as the commitment to my child.

Then I had to leave the candles to burn down while silently chanting, I am ready to love my child, over and over again.

After I smelt the burnt wicks sizzling out, I looked at the next instructions.

Take the bowl and eggshells into the garden with the symbol of your baby and bury them.

I dug a hole at the far end of the garden so Karl wouldn't notice it, then put the baby stuff and eggshells in and poured the contents of the bowl on top of them. I covered it up saying, 'Mother Earth, please accept my symbol of fertility in return for your gift of joy.'

I looked at the final instructions.

Place the drawstring bag with quartz and rosemary under your pillow and await a child to grow inside you without anxiety.

Without anxiety? Hello?

The Taliban Torturer

Next up in my arsenal of relaxation and fertility was yoga. I checked out the classes at our local gym and booked myself in for a beginner to intermediate class at 10 a.m. the next day. As I got dressed in some comfy leggings and a T-shirt I started to look forward to it. Poppy was always going on about how good yoga made her feel. Yep, this would definitely calm me down and stop all the anxiety.

When I arrived, the class was packed full of the blue-rinse brigade. About thirty men and women over the age of sixty-five were standing around chatting like they'd known each other for years. I must've been the youngest one there. Was this OAPs' discount day? Still, they looked a pretty supple bunch.

The teacher, who was about a hundred years old himself, walked to the front of the class. His posture was amazing, straight back, elongated neck, not a slouchy bit in sight. I took note of my own slightly rounded shoulders and pulled them back.

'Hello again, everyone.' He smiled at the crowd.

'Hello,' everyone said with enthusiasm, and one old woman next to me let out a girlish giggle and gave Papa Yogi a coy smile as if she fancied the pants off him.

'OK, let's start with a breathing mantra,' he said. 'Rub your hands together and place them in prayer position with the thumbs pressed into your sternum.'

I did as I was told, liking the sound of breathing exercises. Nothing too strenuous, just nice relaxing deep breaths. Fab.

'We're going to take a deep breath and repeat Sat Nam. Long on the Sat and short on the Nam.' He nodded at everyone to begin.

A collective deep breath took over the room as they all started chanting, 'Saaaaaaaaaaaaaaaaaaaaaaaaaaaaaat Nam.'

'And again,' he said.

I joined in with everyone, not really knowing what it was supposed to do, and feeling a bit embarrassed, but trying to be open to it. If it got rid of all my stress, who cared if I sounded like an injured sheep.

'Now, we'll do the warm-up with Sun Salutations.' Papa Yogi stood up, raising his hands so far behind his head I thought they must be spring loaded, then sweeping them down to the floor and performing a few jumpy press-up type thingies before bouncing back to his feet again. 'And REPEAT!' He ordered.

All the other old biddies were contorting their bodies in positions mine just wouldn't cooperate with. They were bent in half, feet and hands flat on the floor, foreheads pressed against their knees, and I could only get the tips of my fingertips to my knees. But I wasn't going to be beaten. Oh, no! If the oldies could do it, I certainly could.

Now what? I glanced up to see which move they were on next and ouch…crick in my neck!

'And LUNGE…' he shouted.

Everyone inhaled in unison and stepped their right leg back. I got confused between my left and right and had to change it a few times before we were onto Plank pose, which seemed a bit easier, if you were a plank.

A few more laps of the warm up and I was getting more into the swing of things, although I was a bit out of breath, and it reminded me of a TV program I'd watched once about boot camps. I checked out the oldies, who seemed to be breathing perfectly, and they hadn't even broken into a sweat. I grunted and groaned loudly with exertion, much to the annoyance of the people around me who kept glaring at my sudden outbursts. God, if this was the beginners to intermediate class, I dreaded to think what the advanced one was like.

'And HANDS UP!' Papa Yogi jumped to a standing position with his arms in the air, then pressed them back in prayer pose. After all the vigorous bouncing around his next words were like music to me. 'And take a moment to breathe. Nice deep, slow breaths. In and out.'

Oh, yes, I liked this position. Much less strenuous. I tried my best to ignore all the other heavy breathers around me, which sounded like I was in the middle of a dirty conference call on a sex chat line.

Then I attempted to keep up as we flew through various poses called Upward Dog, Cat-Cow, and Downward Dog. Why were they obsessed with animals?

Out of breath, wobbly, and trying to get my body into positions that were just not normal wasn't exactly what I'd call relaxing, but I decided to persevere. Poppy swore by it. Of course I wouldn't be able to manage everything in the first class, but if I carried on, I'd be chilled-out and pregnant in no time.

I found myself in Triangle pose, although I wasn't entirely sure how I'd got there. My right foot was in front of me, the toes pointing forwards, and my left foot way behind with my toes pointing out to the side so I looked like, yep, you guessed it, a triangle. My right hand was supposed to be on my ankle like the other contortionists but I could only get it to just below my knee. And my left hand was attempting to stay up in the air without dropping off from exhaustion.

'And we'll move into Half Moon pose,' Papa Yogi said as I blew the sweaty hair off my forehead to see what he was up to now.

'Slide your right foot forward.'

Forward? Any more forward and I was going to cut myself in half!

'Now place your right hand on the ground, palms flat, and lift your left leg so it's parallel to the floor.'

Well, that was easy for him to say.

I just managed to touch the floor with the tip of my right hand, trying desperately to support my body weight since my left leg was now quivering in the air somewhere behind me. But then I made the mistake of looking at the person next to me to check if I was doing it right, and that caused me to over-wobble, sending me crashing to the floor. I missed the soft landing of the mat, bashed my nose on the hard laminate flooring, and almost ripped my arm out of its socket in the process.

'Unh!' I saw stars and the pain in my nose made my eyes stream.

I rolled on the ground, clutching my nose, partly to make sure it was still in one piece, and partly because if I let it go I knew it would hurt even more.

'Are you OK?' Papa Yogi stood over me as the rest of the OAPs looked on in astonishment.

I pulled my hand away from my nose and there was blood. Lots of blood.

Everyone gasped.

'You're having a nosebleed,' Papa Yogi said, pushing my head back and pinching the bridge of my nose hard.

'Ouch!' I yelped as he squeezed harder. I thought all these yoga people were supposed to be kind and healing. He was more like a Taliban torturer.

He carried on squeezing for about five minutes as the others huffed and puffed and sighed like I'd ruined all their fun.

'How's that?' He finally removed his vice-like pinch.

I put my head forward and waited for blood drips to appear. Nothing. Phew! Although I couldn't say the same for my shoulder, which was now throbbing like it had just been amputated. I shrugged it round in its socket and winced.

'Would you like to carry on?' Papa Yogi asked, although the tone in his voice suggested I should bugger off now before I interrupted even more of their precious time.

Was he joking? No, I would most definitely not be carrying on. This was hardly the relaxing experience I was hoping for.

More Pricks

My temperature hasn't gone up again so I haven't ovulated yet. One more go at sex tonight and then that will be enough for this month. How can I make it more stimulating and exciting? Karl was taking longer and longer to get a stiffy. What if one day he couldn't get it up? Right, thinking cap on. I need to make it more exciting and spontaneous. Even though it's not spontaneous, at all, because we absolutely *have* to do it today in a small slot of time between him getting home, dinner, and Amelia coming round. Maybe I should answer the door naked. No, perhaps not. I'm sure our neighbour across the road caught a sneaky peek the last time I did that.

This was my sixth and final cycle of Clomid, and I couldn't even bring myself to think about what would happen if it didn't work.

My womb is a flower.

Today is my first acupuncture session, and the thought of being pricked with needles is a teensy bit scary. The way I feel at the moment, I've had enough pricks to last me a lifetime!

But it was one of the suggestions Poppy came up with, so I'd been Googling it like mad. Apparently it was good for promoting the circulation of blood in the pelvic cavity, improving ovarian function, and enhancing follicle production. It could also reduce stress levels, and mine were through the roof.

As soon as I entered the Chinese Medicine and Acupuncture Centre a pungent smell of incense and herbs hit me, which made it quite comforting somehow.

'I'm here for an acupuncture session,' I told the tiny Chinese lady behind the counter.

'One minute, please.' She disappeared behind a curtain and came back with an equally tiny Chinese man who looked a bit like Mr Miyagi from *The Karate Kid*.

'Follow me, please.' He took off through a curtain at the side of the counter.

The back of the shop had been set up for treatments, and there were several rooms with couches and incense burning. He led me to one of the rooms and motioned for me to sit down on a chair next to the couch.

After asking me for details of my complaint and general health, he took my pulse in three different areas on each wrist and looked at my tongue while nodding to himself.

A few minutes later, I was up on the couch on my back with needles in my head, neck, legs, and stomach. I looked like that guy out of the *Hellraiser* films.

'Just relax and lie here until I come back. Then I'll take these ones out and put some in your back.'

I thought it would be quite hard to relax with hundreds of needles in you (OK, slight exaggeration, probably twenty-five), but for the first time in ages I felt a calmness wash over me and promptly disappeared into la la land.

Half an hour later, he woke me up, took out the needles and asked me to turn over so he could do my back.

When he left, I thought I'd drop off again, but my brain wouldn't shut up. All I could think about was what we'd do if all the treatments didn't work. Karl hated the thought of IVF. He thought it was messing around with nature somehow. Growing a baby in a test tube wasn't his idea of becoming a dad. Hell, it wasn't exactly the way I saw motherhood, either, and I wasn't looking forward to the possibility of having to go through even more stressful treatments, but if it meant getting pregnant, what choice did I have?

Then what if that didn't work? There were other things we could try. Egg donation, surrogacy, adoption, and I'd checked all of them out on the Internet.

Egg donation still wouldn't guarantee a successful outcome, and Karl was worried that we wouldn't know anything about the mother's genes. I replayed a conversation in my head that we'd had a while ago...

'What if the baby grew up to be a serial killer?' he said. 'The mum could be a complete nutter for all we know.'

'All donors are screened for any health problems and have a psychological evaluation before they're allowed to donate,' I said. 'They won't let any nutters in.'

'Yes, but how do we know for sure?'

I shrugged. 'Do you ever know with your own children what will happen? Who knows what quirks or genes you might pass down to your kids? I mean, look at your cousin Jamie who's a kleptomaniac.'

'That was a misunderstanding. He's a diabetic and his blood sugar was really low so he needed to eat some chocolate quickly. That's the only reason he took it from the shop.'

'What, a hundred times, from shops all over the London area?' I raised a disbelieving eyebrow.

'Well, stealing a few bars of chocolate isn't exactly on a par with being a nutter.'

'Adoption is another option,' I huffed. Although it could take longer than six months to be approved, and then God knows how long to actually find a child. There weren't enough babies to go around, so we would either have to consider an older child, who would no doubt have a whole host of psychological problems by being separated from its parents, or consider adopting a baby from abroad. The possible complications of adoption were pretty scary.

'What about Graham Beange?' Karl nodded knowingly at me. 'He was adopted and murdered his dad. There was a big study done years ago into the amount of killers who'd been adopted at birth.'

I sighed, feeling miffed that he seemed to be putting obstacles in the way. 'You're obsessed with killers!'

'What about Sandra Bridewell a.k.a The Black Widow. She killed three husbands, and she was adopted,' he said.

'Yes, I can understand that sometimes! Sometimes I'd like to kill mine.' I rolled my eyes at him. 'Not every child who's adopted will turn out to be a killer. That's ridiculous.'

'But my point is, you just don't know, do you? Most of the children will have lots of social, psychological, and health issues from being abandoned. That won't be easy to cope with. And I very much doubt we'd be lucky enough to get a baby, which would mean adopting one from abroad, and that brings a whole host of other problems.

'Yes, but what about…' I wracked my brains, trying to come up with a counter-argument. 'Madonna! She's adopted and all her kids seem to be fine. And Angelina and Brad. They adopted loads of kids. If it's good enough for them, it should be good enough for us,' I said smugly.

'We need to do some more research on it before we have a proper discussion.'

'There's surrogacy, too. Your sperm is OK, so you could fertilise another woman, and she could carry our baby.' I decided to ignore his negativity.

'Oh, wow, you mean I get to have sex with another woman?' He winked at me. 'Are there any hot babes that do it?'

'Ha! You wish!' I raised an eyebrow.

He paused for a moment, thinking, maybe about hot babes. 'What about that case in the papers a while ago?'

'What case?'

'A couple made an agreement with a surrogate, and then she decided halfway through the pregnancy that she wanted to keep the child. They'd already handed over five grand in expenses, and then the court ruled that the surrogate could keep the baby *and* the couple would have to pay her child support!'

'Oh, for God's sake! Anyone would think you didn't want a baby,' I snapped.

His face softened. 'Of course I do. It's just that there are a lot of issues to consider if your treatment doesn't work. And with surrogacy, it's not like you can choose the perfect woman with the perfect genes to have a baby with. I already have the perfect woman.' He smiled at me. 'With surrogacy we'd be dealing with limited options. The baby wouldn't have your genes, or your feisty spirit.'

OK, so maybe it was the voice of reason, and maybe it was true. I just didn't want to think about it.

Half an hour later, Mr Miyagi arrived to remove the needles. 'I'd like you to come once a week. And it would also be beneficial to give you some Chinese herbs to increase your fertility,' he said.

'OK.' I followed him back into the shop as he set about mixing various things in individual paper bags. It looked like a concoction of dried bark, leaves, and goat's poo.

Ew. I hoped it tasted better than it looked.

He handed me the bags. 'Boil these into a tea and drink them twice a day.'

As soon as I got home I boiled up the compost-looking herbs. The smell as they bubbled away was gross.

I took one sip and heaved. I tried again and managed to get a little bit down, although it was threatening to come back up pretty quick. Blah! It was like drinking boiled up sumo wrestlers' jock straps. No wonder you never saw a fat Chinese person if this was what they had to drink.

I poured the tea down the sink and chucked the rest of the herbs in a kitchen cupboard. Maybe I'd just stick with the acupuncture instead.

Getting Pregnant is Like Wanting a PlayStation

I didn't think about babies for four whole hours today, which must've been a record. And that was only because I didn't turn on the TV to be bombarded with adverts for baby stuff, I didn't go out of the house to see happy mothers pushing their babies along the street with glowing smiles on their faces, and I didn't have any clients who had children they wanted to talk about.

Instead, I scrubbed the house from top to bottom. It was way overdue for a spring clean anyway, and it did actually help to get my mind off things for a while.

Well, that was until Wicked Stepmother phoned up. Groan. I'm surprised she needs a phone when she's a witch and could use telepathy or a spell to annoy me instead.

'Ah, Gina,' she trilled.

'Hello, Lavinia. How are you?' I tried to sound pleased to hear from her, but wasn't sure if she was buying it.

'Let me get straight to the point,' she said in a brusque voice. No change there, then. No "Hello, how are you, Gina? What have you been up to?" Oh, no, the only people Lavinia thought about were herself and her equally selfish daughter. 'It's Jayne and Wayne's wedding anniversary tonight and I wanted to ask if you could baby-sit for them. The au pair has suddenly left them in the lurch.'

The first thing I did was laugh to myself about the Jayne and Wayne reference. Next, I cringed. I didn't really want to be around any kids at the moment. It sounds strange when you desperately want them yourself, but it's a constant reminder of your problems. It was bad enough seeing Kerry, who was now showing her beautiful baby bump. And why couldn't Jayne ask me herself?

'Um...' I wondered if I could come up with an excuse in one second. Think! 'OK,' I replied when my brain-wracking didn't work. *Shit.*

'Good. Your father and I are going out for a meal with them,' she rattled off quickly.

'How nice,' I muttered, wondering why anyone in their right minds would want Lavinia tagging along on their wedding anniversary celebrations.

'Well, that's all settled, then. We have a table booked at Rosita's at eight, so I'll expect you at their house around seven-fifteen,' she said, all business-like.

'OK. How's Dad?' I asked, and then realized I was listening to the dialling tone.

I stared at the phone in my hand, not really believing she'd just done that. And not even a mention of how the fertility treatment was going. Still, why should I expect her to be any different? She'd been the same ever since she performed some kind of voodoo and swept my dad under her spell. Why couldn't I stand up to her?

We arrived at Jayne and Wayne's six-bedroomed mansion on the dot and Lavinia still moaned at us for being late. I walked into their newly refurbished kitchen that was practically as big as the whole downstairs floor area of my house. It gleamed and sparkled with new appliances yet to be used. The place was immaculate, and I knew for a fact Jayne didn't have either the time or the inclination to get a mop and bucket out. The poor au pair would be worked to death, which was why there always seemed to be a high turnover of them in this household.

With two energetic boys, it was unnatural for the place to be so clinically neat and tidy, and I'd seen Jayne and Wayne (ha ha!) telling the boys off if they so much as left a crumb on the top-of-the-range shiny marble breakfast bar. If I ever became a parent there is no way I'd want to stifle their

116

natural urges to explore and play and have fun in their own environment by turning it into a show house for *Ideal Home* magazine. I wondered if Rupert and Quentin would grow up with an obsessive-compulsive disorder about cleanliness or, even worse, turn into serial killers from lack of cuddles and nurturing.

The boys were running around upstairs in their bedroom, screaming and shouting like they'd just had too many E numbers, and for once, Jayne and Wayne didn't seem to care. Knowing them, they'd probably plied Rupert and Quentin with loads of fizzy drinks and chocolate bars just to get back at me.

'Where's Dad?' I asked.

'In the toilet.' Lavinia crinkled up her nose, obviously finding the T-word distasteful. 'Honestly, I'm always waiting for him. That man is so selfish sometimes.' She smoothed down her glossy chignon.

Him, selfish? Oooh, the woman had a bloody cheek! I clamped my mouth shut before I said something I'd regret.

'No baby yet, then?' Lavinia eyed my flat stomach.

'No,' I grumbled.

'Well, stop being so impatient. Honestly, you youngsters today are in such a hurry to do everything.' Lavinia frowned.

'I'm not being impatient,' I huffed. 'I've been trying for eighteen months and I'm not getting anywhere!'

Karl sloped off to see the boys before he could get a Lavinia-bashing as well.

Jayne nodded her agreement in the background as Wayne mumbled something about bringing the boys downstairs and made a sharp exit, too.

'You should make the most of it while you can. Once you have them, you'll never have any freedom, and life will never be the same again.' Jayne waved a dismissive hand.

I stood, hand on hip. 'Of course it's not going to be the same again! That's the whole point, isn't it? I don't want my life to be the same. I *want* to feel the unconditional, maternal love when I hold my baby for the first time and realize what

117

an incredible miracle it is.' I glared at Jayne, who probably didn't have a clue what I was talking about since she didn't seem to have a maternal bone in her body. 'What I'd give up by losing my so-called *freedom* wouldn't even compare to the joy and excitement of being a parent,' I snapped, reaching boiling point now. 'You should try it some time.' Ew! How did she even have the nerve to complain about her wonderful boys when she was lucky enough to have them in the first place?

Jayne gasped and crossed her arms defensively. 'And what would you know about it, seeing as you can't seem to get pregnant?' She arched a superior eyebrow. 'Being a mother isn't always a bed of roses.'

'Of course it's not, but I want to experience *all* of motherhood. The highs *and* the lows. It's the most important job in the world.'

Jayne snorted. 'No, being a barrister and trying high-profile murder cases is the most important job in the world. Being a parent is damned hard work with very little reward, and it's not a proper job.'

'Well, I guess that all boils down to your priorities in life,' I said with disgust, narrowing my eyes at the selfish cow.

'I hope you're not always this snappy and grumpy.' Lavinia raised a perfectly shaped eyebrow at me (an eyebrow, I hasten to add, that she didn't get me to wax. Oh, no, instead she'd rather take her business to Pamper Me in the high street. Maybe supporting your family wasn't in the Witches Codebook of Ethics). 'Karl will get fed up with you and have an affair if you're not careful.' She wagged her French-manicured finger at me (yep, Pamper Me again!).

'Well, thanks a lot for that cheery little thought, Lavinia,' I said, desperately trying hard to fight the urge to stab both of them with my high-heeled boot.

Lavinia stood, scrutinizing me. 'And look at the state of you. You've really let yourself go. Your hair needs a wash, your skin is pale and blotchy. Not a very good advert for a beauty business, is it?' She let out a loud tut and ran a hand through her immaculate hair again to ram the point home. 'Mark my words, young lady. Get a grip of yourself before Karl leaves you. No man appreciates a nagging, highly strung moaner,' she said, conveniently forgetting that those words described her to a T.

I rolled my eyes at her, about to let them both have it, when the boys both yelled and ran into me like a couple of out-of-control rockets, hugging me around the waist, thankfully ending the rant from Lavinia. 'Aunty Ginaaaaaaaaaaaaaaaaaa!'

Karl appeared and we were bombarded with questions.

'What are we going to play tonight?'

'How long are you here for?'

'Are you staying until tomorrow?'

'What about Cluedo?'

'Can we play cards?'

'Rupert, Quentin, come along now. Sit down and behave for your Aunty Gina and Uncle Karl,' Jayne said with a wicked glint in her eye, probably hoping they would do neither.

Rupert and Quentin looked at each other and, surprisingly, sat down quietly like a pair of little choirboys.

'How are you, love?' Dad crept up behind me and put a hand on my shoulder as the others left and got in the car. I hoped he hadn't heard my little outburst earlier. As much as I didn't particularly get on with Lavinia and Jayne, I didn't want Dad to be in the middle of a family feud.

I gave him a half-hearted smile.

'You're looking tired.' He rubbed my shoulder.

'Well, all this fertility stuff is taking its toll. This is the last month of the Clomid. I should find out any day whether it's worked or not.'

He gave my shoulder a reassuring squeeze. 'Just think positive.'

I looked up glumly. 'It's not easy. If it doesn't work, we'll have to try IVF.'

'I'm sure everything will work out in the end,' Dad said as

Lavinia poked her perfectly coiffed head through the door.

'Come on! You're lagging behind, as usual.' She threw him a disapproving look.

He turned to face her, a flash of anger in his eyes. 'I'm talking to my daughter, and if you have to wait an extra five minutes then so be it. Unlike you and Jayne, I *do* consider parenting to be the most important job in the world.'

Yay! Go Dad!

A red flush crept up Lavinia's neck and she disappeared back outside.

'Women!' Dad shook his head, then hugged me and smiled fondly at Karl before slipping out the door to enjoy a night of covens and spells.

I looked at Rupert and Quentin, who were sitting at the kitchen table like little cherubs, eyeing the Cluedo board with excitement.

'OK,' Karl said, taking off his coat and rolling his sleeves up. 'We're in for a fun-fest, little guys.'

We sat down opposite Rupert and Quentin and got out the board.

'Can I be Captain Peacock?' Quentin asked.

'I want to be Colonel Mustard!' Rupert said.

'You can be anyone you want to be.' I grinned, dishing out the pieces.

An hour later, we were on to Monopoly. Karl had his arm draped around Quentin, explaining the finer points of why he should buy the expensive Mayfair. Their heads were close together as Quentin looked up at Karl with hero-worship adoration. Karl ruffled his hair and they gave each other a high five.

My stomach clenched. He would make such a good dad it almost broke my heart to see it. I could clearly picture him kicking a football around with our little boy for hours on end; see him running around the garden with our son on his shoulders, who was squealing with delight. And if we had a girl, I envisioned him holding onto her hand for dear life as she took her first steps, or taking her to dancing lessons, sitting in the front row of her dance recitals, cheering her on.

'We never get to play games with Mummy and Daddy,' Rupert's voice broke into my daydream. 'They're always too busy.'

Quentin looked up at me with huge eyes and a wistful smile. 'I wish you were our parents. You're so much fun.'

'Well, if we were your parents, we wouldn't have as much fun time to spend with you like we do now,' I said, defending Jayne and Wayne (ha ha!), because it seemed like the right thing to do.

'But you never tell us off,' Rupert said.

Karl and I both chuckled.

'That's because we're your aunty and uncle,' Karl said. 'If we were your parents, we would tell you off sometimes, too. It's different when you all live together. Sometimes we get on each other's nerves when we live with each other. Gina definitely gets on my nerves sometimes.' He raised an eyebrow at me and grinned.

'Hey!' I gave him a playful swat across the arm. 'Uncle Karl is right. When you're an aunty or grandparent, you get to spend fun time with each other. Parents have the hard job.' I swallowed to stop the tears forming.

'But Granny Lavinia is so bossy. We don't get to spend fun time with her, either.'

I was taking a sip of chamomile tea at the time and nearly splurted it out with laughter. I bet Lavinia wouldn't like being called Granny.

'Why aren't you a mummy?' Rupert looked up at me.

'I…well…' I could feel the tears threatening to burst. I glanced away so they wouldn't see I was upset.

Karl put his arm around my shoulder. 'It's not always easy for people to be parents,' he said to them, his voice cracking on the last word.

I grabbed his other hand and squeezed it. He squeezed back.

'Sometimes in life, no matter how much we might want something, it doesn't happen,' Karl said.

'What, like when I wanted a PlayStation for Christmas and I didn't get it?' Quentin asked.

Despite myself, I did smile at that. If only it could be that simple.

'Something like that,' I said, holding my arms out for a hug. They both rushed over to get an Aunty Gina special cuddle.

I rested my head on the top of theirs, kissing their hair, which smelt of shampoo and little boys, and I didn't want to let them go.

Five hours later, my period arrived.

Decisions, Decisions

Eight days later, I was sitting in Dr Dye's office again. The model fufu had been relegated to the shelf at the back of his desk. Maybe someone had used it as an offensive weapon, after all.

'Well, the next option is IVF,' he said.

I nodded vigorously. 'Yes, I know that. I want to start as soon as possible.'

'We don't carry out IVF in this clinic, but there are plenty of fantastic facilities available. You can be referred for two IVF treatments through the National Health Service, and the waiting list for that is at least a couple of years. Or, you can be referred as a private patient to a fertility clinic or hospital.'

More nodding. 'Yes, we'd like to go private. Can you suggest anywhere? Where's the best one? What are the chances of getting pregnant? How long will it take?' I rattled off.

He held his hands up with a slight smile to fight off my bombarding questions. 'It will be up to you to choose a clinic. You can look on the Internet and research which one suits you best. There's plenty of information available to help you choose. Some clinics have a better success rate than others, so that's something you'll need to consider. You'll also have to think about location. There will be numerous scans and appointments during the treatment so you'll want to be fairly local to the clinic, unless you're going to stay somewhere close by.' He pulled out some headed paper and started scribbling. 'I'll write you a referral letter to take with you.' He handed it to me.

I took it, trying to make out what is said. Did all doctors have to pass a class in gobbledygook, random scribbling before they passed their exams? I peered at the scrawl harder, pretty sure I could make out the words, "ostrich," "kebab," "football," and something that looked Chinese. No wonder there were cases of people having the wrong body parts operated on. How would anyone have a clue what the doctors' notes said? Scary!

'And here's a website address that will be helpful for you.' Another random scribbling.

I took that, too, but at least it was legible. 'Right.' I stood up, feeling a sudden gravity pull towards my PC and Google. I put my hand out to shake his.

'Good luck,' he said.

'Thanks.'

'Oh, and Gina,' he said as I was swinging his door open. 'Just relax and be positive.'

Grrrrrrrrrrrrrrrrrrrrr.

Armed with a green tea, I switched on the computer. My first stop was the website Dr Dye had given me of the HFEA, who are the governing body for fertility treatment. It had a really nifty search facility to check out success rates of treatments and the location of the clinics. I decided to look in the London area because we were in easy reach of the train station. And since it only took half an hour to get to King's Cross, I figured another half an hour on the tube and I could probably be there, so London clinics worked out the closest.

Next, I looked at success rates of live births from IVF. The majority of them were around an average of 30% for women under thirty-five, and I just fell into that category.

30 percent? Yikes! That was so low.

I sat back in the chair, staring at the screen, checking and double-checking to make sure I'd got that right. Yep, I had.

I always thought IVF had a really high success rate, so this was a shock to me.

God, the odds weren't looking good.

I narrowed it down to two clinics and then checked their waiting times. Even though I was going private, there was still a big queue of hopeful couples out there. One of the clinics had a waiting time of five months. The other was three months. Two months was an eternity in the life of a desperate, infertile woman, so I phoned the latter – Guy's and St Thomas' Assisted Conception Unit.

'Hi, I'd like to book an appointment to start IVF treatment,' I told the girl who answered the phone.

'OK, if you can just give me your details, please. Name and address?'

I rattled them off.

'Doctor's details.'

'Dr Dye.'

I couldn't be sure but I think she suppressed a snort.

'Are you NHS or self-funding?' she asked.

'Self-funding.'

'And what fertility treatment have you had to date?'

I told her everything that had happened in the last eighteen months. God, had it really been that long? What if another eighteen months went by and I was still childless?

No. Be positive, Gina. This will work.

'So when can I make an appointment to see a consultant?' I asked.

'First, I need to send you out an information pack with a list of fees and a questionnaire. When we get that back, we'll allocate you onto our next patient information evening, which explains all aspects of treatments.'

Oh, God. More waiting? 'Can't I just make an appointment now? Do we have to go to the information evening?'

'I'm afraid so,' she said in a sympathetic tone. 'IVF is very demanding, both mentally and physically, and we want to make sure all prospective patients understand the treatment cycles in detail.'

I let out a small huff. 'When's the next one?'

'Three weeks. I tell you what, I'll pencil you in for that

125

date, and when we get the forms back, I'll send you a confirmation letter.'

'Great! What date is that?'

She told me and I marked it on the calendar that I was sick of looking at. Three whole weeks.

Karl and I lay in bed that night, me with my head on his shoulder, curled up in the crook of his arm, Karl gently stroking my back.

'A thirty percent chance of success is nothing.' I stared through the darkness at the ceiling as thoughts about the IVF whizzed through my head like a tornado.

He sighed.

I glanced up at him. 'What?'

'For once, can't we have a conversation that doesn't revolve around having a baby?'

I tutted. What else was there to talk about? This was the most important thing in the world.

We were silent for a few minutes.

'It's just that this is really important so we need to talk about it.' I carried on anyway. 'I mean, thirty percent? I still can't get my head round that.'

He groaned, knowing I wasn't going to shut up. 'It's better than, say, a five percent chance.'

'What if it doesn't work?' I gnawed on my bottom lip, thinking about the prospect.

'Stop being negative. You need to think more positive, Gina. If you think it won't work, then it won't. It'll be like a self-fulfilling prophecy.'

'You're right. It will work. It will work. It *will* work,' I said.

'That's more like it.' He kissed my forehead.

'But what if it doesn't?'

'Gina!'

'What?' I said in mock surprise.

'Shut up. I've got a busy day at work tomorrow and I need some sleep. Stop over-analyzing every little thing all the time.'

As he turned over, I sent a silent message to Zelda. Maybe she'd talk to me.

Hey, Zelda! Are you awake?

Nothing.

Pssssst. Zelda, can you send me a sign that this is going to work? Go on, just an itsy bitsy sign to let me know. If you've got time, of course. I know you're probably busy out doing Universey things. Go on. I'll do anything you want in return.

Still nothing. Not a squeak in the floorboards or a rattle in the central heating pipes as an acknowledgement.

Look, here's the thing. I know I've been a hyper, impatient, slightly insane pain in the arse lately, but I just want this so badly. Soooooooo badly. And I deserve to be a mother. I'd make a great mum. Karl would make a fabulous dad. So if you can send me a sign that it will work then I'll be able to relax like everyone keeps telling me.

P.S. Did I mention how badly I want this?

Zelda?

Finding the Balance

The next day, the letter from Guy's arrived through the letterbox, along with a leaflet that had been stuffed through. I ignored the leaflet, putting it to one side, and tore open the brown A4 envelope. Inside was a brochure, a list of fees, and the questionnaire.

I scoured the brochure which listed the fertility treatments they carried out – IVF, ICSI, sperm retrieval, donor eggs – how to optimize your chances of getting pregnant by eating healthily and taking folic acid (yep, knew all about that bit), and the side effects of treatment:

24% of treatments which resulted in pregnancy end in miscarriage.

What? You mean I could go through it all, get pregnant, and then lose the baby anyway? Why are there so many obstacles in the way? I thought modern technology was so advanced these days.

Ovarian hyperstimulation syndrome, which causes the ovaries to enlarge and blood oestrogen levels to rise. Symptoms include abdominal swelling and bloating.

Oooh, that sounds fun!

Ectopic pregnancies.

God!

Pelvic infection from egg collection.

Something else to look forward to.

Bleeding. There is a small chance the needle passed through the vagina for egg collection could puncture the bowel.

Great!

Drug side effects.

You mean you turn into a raging, hormonal nutter. Oh, yeah, been there, done that!

Foetal abnormality. There is evidence that IVF/ICSI babies are more likely to be born prematurely.

Maybe I should give it all up now. Maybe we just aren't supposed to be parents. Or is this supposed to be some sort of journey I'm meant to take? Do I have to prove something first? And if so, what? Is it supposed to be a lesson teaching me something valuable to pass on to my kids?

I read it all and felt sick. It sounded horrendous. And, even worse, the chances of it working were pretty slim. I had a 30% chance of getting pregnant, with a possible 24% chance of having a miscarriage if I did. All that and we'd have to pay three thousand pounds to go through it.

But what choice did I have? It was my only hope. It was my final weapon in the infertility war.

I filled out the questionnaire with a heavy heart, stuck it in an envelope and stomped down the road to post it. Then I thought maybe I shouldn't be sending it off with such negative vibes so I kissed the back of the envelope and made a wish. Feeling sorry for myself wasn't going to help anything.

Please work.

I ignored the pink lip gloss marks on it, took a deep breath, and shoved it in the post box.

When I came back home I glanced at the leaflet that had arrived…

New to the area, Suzanne Fielder – Energy Crystal Healing Practitioner

What is Energy Crystal Healing?

129

Energy Healing is a wonderful non-invasive holistic therapy, which means that the focus is on the individual as a whole, rather than on physical symptoms alone. The aim is to restore wholeness, balance, and health to emotions, mind and spirit, as well as the physical body.

Our Energy Centres within the body and our Energy Field (or Aura) that surrounds us can become blocked or imbalanced, causing illness or upset to our system. Energy Healing, incorporating Crystals, Colour Breathing, and Meditation techniques can help to release these mental and physical blockages, allowing the body to heal.

Crystal therapy is effective in treating stress, anxiety, insomnia, depression, menstrual disorders, reproductive system imbalances (infertility, PCOS, and supports IVF treatment), muscular pain, digestive problems, and many more.

Find the balance you need...

I knew it sounded like something whacky and bizarre that Poppy would come out with, and I didn't know exactly how this was going to help me, but, more importantly, it sounded pretty damn likely it could be a message from Zelda, telling me this woman could help me make the IVF work. My heart broke into a tap-dancing beat and a surge of adrenaline shot through me.

I scanned the leaflet again, devouring it with my eyes. Yep, I was sure this was meant for me.

'Oh, my God, you'll never guess what!' I told Poppy on the phone, and carried on without pausing for breath. 'You were right! I think Zel...I mean, the Universe answered one of my questions.'

'Hey, that's great!' she said. 'What happened?'

I filled her in on the leaflet. 'So, I think that's what she was trying to tell me. Somehow, and I don't know how, I think this crystal healing woman will help the IVF to work.'

'You know, I was going to mention crystal healing to you, but I knew there wasn't a practitioner local to you. It's all about balancing yourself, getting inspiration from within to make you calmer.'

'Well, it's amazing because this woman has just moved to the area! If that's not a sign, then I don't know what is.'

'So when are you going to see her?'

'Well, Karl will think I've completely lost the plot if I go and see someone like that. He doesn't believe in all that "mumbo jumbo." But I'm going to give her a ring now. No time like the present!' I had a good feeling about this. OK, so I thought that every time I tried something new. Although I'd done the feng shui and yoga, there must be a reason why people said third time lucky, mustn't there? It would work. It had to.

Later that afternoon, I was knocking on Suzanne's door. Luckily, as she was new to the area, she wasn't booked up. I expected her to be older and frumpy and wearing a flowery muumuu. But no, she was in her early forties, trendy, with really kind eyes.

'Hi!' She gave me a friendly smile and I felt instantly at ease with her. 'Come in, come in. I've just moved in so I'm still unpacking.' She nodded to some boxes stacked up in the hallway under the stairs.

'Oh, I know what you mean. We moved into our house five years ago, and we still haven't unpacked everything,' I said.

'Follow me into the treatment room.' She led me up the stairs, along a light and airy corridor to a room at the end.

The interior was warm, cosy, and inviting. Dimmed lights with scented candles, a soft blanket on the treatment couch, and various beautifully coloured crystals everywhere.

'Have a seat on the couch,' she said, perching on the end of a wooden stool. 'Have you ever had crystal healing before?'

I shook my head, for some reason feeling slightly ridiculous.

She gave me a warm smile. 'Let me explain a little bit about it, then we'll talk about you, and why you're here, and I'll carry out a healing therapy designed especially for you.'

'OK.' My shoulders relaxed.

'Crystal therapy is an ancient holistic treatment that works on the whole body, not just any symptoms you might have. It helps you to get well naturally by relaxing and re-energising you, and getting rid of any physical and emotional blockages you might have.'

I nodded. I could definitely do with relaxing, and if it could unblock my fufu, then great!

She handed me a pink, smooth crystal. 'Crystals have obviously been around for millions of years, and the human body is crystalline in nature, so they affect our bodies at an energetic level to promote healing. They contain universal energy and each one has different healing properties or forces to raise your energy field.'

I caressed the crystal in my hand. 'Sounds good to me.'

She tilted her head, studying me for a few minutes. 'What problems are you having?'

I glanced down at the floor for a second before answering. 'I'm having problems getting pregnant.' I filled her in on everything that had happened so far.

She listened and nodded slowly. Then she reached out her warm hand and placed it over mine. 'Crystal therapy is an excellent treatment that can complement fertility drugs and IVF. And the good thing about it is that it's naturally calming. When you don't feel whole, mentally or physically, your body tenses up and can restrict blood and oxygen flow throughout, including your ovaries. Women who go through fertility problems are often storing negative emotions like anger, fear, jealousy, and depression, which create energy blockages in your chakras and can manifest in real physical and mental problems.'

I felt a chill go through me. She was absolutely right. I had been feeling like that. I thought it was just me going crazy, or turning into someone I didn't recognize, but maybe this was natural for a lot of women in the same situation. At last, someone understood exactly what I was going through, and that seemed to put me instantly at ease.

'OK, if you lie down and take off your shoes, I'm going to spend a moment tuning into you,' she said.

I kicked off my shoes and swung up onto the couch.

She placed her hands lightly on my feet and closed her eyes. Then she got a white crystal pendulum, holding it over different parts of my body. 'Your base chakra is blocked. This area deals with things like fear and resentment about the baby you want. It's also about living in the moment. All of us live such stressful lives these days. We juggle jobs, chores, busy lives, and are bombarded by more and more distractions. I feel you aren't living in the moment at all. You're constantly waiting for the next thing to happen, and the next, to achieve your goal. And in doing that, you're not enjoying your life, and you're missing the magic around you.'

'Yes, that is so right.' I suddenly felt a tear spring into my eye. 'I feel like I'm living in limbo all the time, just waiting to get pregnant.'

'We need to focus on getting rid of dead energy and negativity in this area.' She moved the pendulum up higher. 'This is your sacral chakra, which is also blocked. This is connected to emotions and fertility. It's the area where your grief is stored.'

No wonder it was blocked.

'And this is your navel chakra. Again, it's blocked. This is about anger and self-esteem. How you project and achieve anything in your life depends on balance in this chakra.' She moved the pendulum higher. 'Your heart chakra is also blocked.'

'Oh, God, I'm not doing very well, am I?' I said.

'Don't worry. This is what you're here to fix. This chakra is about trust, love, and forgiveness. You need to trust in other people and the Universe that you will achieve what you want.'

That tallied up with what Poppy was always telling me.

As Suzanne went through the other chakras they were all blocked.

'You can't switch off.' She smiled at me.

I rolled my eyes in agreement. 'I know.'

'You need to trust again that things will happen and take time to live in the moment to appreciate what you already have. Really believe and have confidence that you will achieve everything you want to in life. Project it out to the Universe. See it in your mind and really visualize it. Think about your motives for wanting it. Think how having a baby will enhance your life. You need to imagine it in your head and use your senses to bring it to life. Hear your baby laughing, see it smiling, smell its hair. And then, let go of it. Because if you know it *will* happen, then it will, and no negativity can hold you back. Trust that if it's meant to be, it will happen.'

'Yes, that makes sense when you say it, but it's easier said than done,' I said.

She let out a soft laugh. 'No one said it would be easy, but you can do it. When you make it clear what you want, the Universe will find a way to give it to you. You just have to have faith, Gina. If you get too stressed about it, the negative energies can block the thing you want most of all.' I thought about that for a moment until she said, 'I can unblock your chakras, but you are your own guru. You are the one with the energy inside you to heal yourself. You just have to believe, and look for signs that will guide you along the way.'

I took a deep breath, feeling my eyes well up in an enlightening, emotional moment. What she said made perfect sense, although Karl would think she was kooky and crazy, since he didn't believe in all this sort of stuff. But somehow, her words brought a shiver up my spine and a tingling inside me. I would try my hardest to do what she said.

'Try repeating a mantra to yourself every day.'

'Oh, I've been doing that already. I've been saying, "My womb is a flower."'

'Good. The more you do it, the more you'll believe it. Leave post-it notes with positive mantras around the house so you can see them every day. That will help you believe this will really happen for you.'

'Good idea.' I made a mental note to do that as soon as I got back.

'Good. Now, I'm going to place some crystals on different parts of your body, so just lie there and relax. You might see images come into your mind, or colours, and that's all normal.'

I closed my eyes and felt her lightly placing the crystals on me. Within a few minutes I was so relaxed I was about to drop off. I peeked an eye open to see what she was doing. With her eyes closed, she had her hands above different parts of my body. My eye drooped shut again and I saw a rainbow of colours behind my lids. Yellow, orange, blue, purple, red. I felt myself fill with a lightness and happiness I'd never experienced before.

Frankenstein's Monster

A few weeks later, we were getting ready for the hospital opening evening. Even though we weren't being judged on what we looked like, I felt like it was a good idea to look smart and make a good impression.

I'd already tried on eight different outfits and nothing seemed right. What if they refused to treat us because we didn't look like parent material? Should I wear something frumpy and boring that showed a practical parent trait? Or should I wear something fashionable that showed I could blend in and conform to society? How about something original to prove I could be a creative mum?

'It's not a fashion show.' Karl eyed the pile of clothes gathering on the bed as he chose the nearest thing in his wardrobe to wear. 'There will probably be so many people there, they won't even have time to notice what you're wearing.'

I zipped up a pair of tight black trousers and tugged on a white blouse. Surely I couldn't go wrong with a simple black and white ensemble.

I was just putting the finishing touches to my mascara in the dressing table mirror when my eyes strayed to the numerous post-it notes I'd put up: *I will get pregnant. Don't worry. Everything will be OK. Zelda, I'm projecting positive baby thoughts.* Karl had written his own and stuck them next to mine. *Who the fuck is Zelda? Can I have a beer yet? My husband is the sexiest guy, ever!*

I'd been trying to put in place everything that Suzanne had suggested about projecting positive thoughts – knowing it would happen, and then forgetting about it – but it was pretty hard to do when you had to change the mind-set and personality you've had since you were born. I'd even bought a crisicola crystal bracelet to wear, and a rose quartz crystal, which I was now wearing down my knickers every day. Apparently, both of them were good for increasing fertility. At least I was trying.

Oh, and speaking of knickers, I'd just gone out and bought twenty orange pairs, since, according to Suzanne, orange was the colour of my sexual chakra. If orange knickers equated to an unblocked fufu chakra then I'd be wearing them twenty-four-seven, even though they looked pretty icky.

'Come on, we're going to miss the train.' Karl glanced at his watch.

'I will get pregnant,' I whispered to myself one more time.

The lecture theatre at the hospital was packed when we arrived. I gripped Karl's hand and we made our way to a couple of empty seats at the front. As we sat down, I glanced around and studied all the other wannabe parents. I could see the strain on their faces that probably mirrored my own. How long had they been trying?

The lights dimmed and a hush of anticipation crackled in the air. A middle-aged man who looked a bit like Herman Munster entered the podium, which was a tad scary.

Karl elbowed me with a horrified look.

My brain went off at a tangent, imagining being strapped to a stretcher by Herman and his best mate Frankenstein in the basement of a dark, damp Victorian hospital. I was screaming as they advanced with lumbering steps to implant me with all sorts of genetically modified embryos that were clones of themselves and they were going to use to take over the world. I'd just got to the part where they got a giant needle out when Herman started talking, sending me spiralling back to reality with a bump.

He explained he was the director of the Assisted Conception Unit, and would be talking us through the fertility treatments they provided so we were all completely sure we wanted to go ahead with it. They would give us statistics on success and failure rates, and advise us what complications there might be.

Since I'd already spent a lifetime online researching IVF, I had a pretty good idea of what it all entailed, but Karl and some of the others looked worried, although I'm not sure if that was because they were imagining the same Herman scenarios as me and thinking that he'd be messing around with their genes to make designer babies or Frankenstein clones.

There was no doubt about it, along with the physical side of things with all the drugs, the mental side sounded equally horrible and demanding. I just hoped Suzanne would be able to help me cope with the stress and frustration of it all.

Two hours later, when the lights went up, I glanced at Karl again, only to find him with his head resting on the shoulder of some poor woman, fast-a-bloody-sleep.

I elbowed him hard in the ribs and he woke up with a start.

'How could you fall asleep?' I hissed.

'I'm tired. I've had a busy week at work,' he whispered.

'Didn't you hear the bit about the low success rates?'

'Of course, I did.'

I folded my arms, watching him carefully. 'What did they say, then?'

'Er…they said we had a thirty percent success rate.'

'You're only saying that because I told you the same thing the other night.'

'Stop worrying, Gina. It will work.' He gave me an encouraging wink.

As we filed out, several members of staff were handing out letters to everyone with their respective first appointment dates. Ours was in four weeks.

On the way out there were coffee, tea, water, and biscuits laid out. Some of the couples hung around to chat to each other.

A skinny couple helped themselves to coffee in the queue

in front of us.

'Oh, great, they've got green tea,' I nudged Karl.

Skinny Girl turned around and smiled at me. 'You're on the green tea, too?'

I nodded. 'Yes, although I draw the line at drinking wee.'

She pointed at me, grinning. 'That weird tribe in Africa, right? Yeah, I read about them, too. Can't say I've tried that one myself yet.'

'No. Yuck.' I grimaced.

'How long have you been trying to get pregnant?' Skinny Guy asked us.

'Nearly two years,' I said, realizing how weird it was that instead of introducing ourselves first, we struck up a conversation based on how long we'd been trying for a baby. In some ways, it was reassuring to know there were so many people out there in the same boat, but in another way, it was even more depressing.

'Five years for us,' Skinny Girl said with a grim smile. 'IVF's our last hope.'

Five years? Five years of intolerable waiting. Five years of fertility purgatory. Two years already felt like five thousand. What would five years feel like?

'Are you worried about Herman Munster running the show?' I asked. 'I'm nervous enough about the IVF already, and he kind of freaked me out a bit.'

Karl chuckled.

Skinny Girl rolled her eyes at me. 'That's just what I was saying to my husband.' She jerked her head in Skinny Guy's direction. 'Wasn't it?'

Skinny Guy nodded.

I did a mock shiver. 'Creepy.'

'I know!' Skinny Girl said. 'Still, they've got one of the best success rates in the country.'

'It's nice to meet someone going through the same thing,' I said, suddenly feeling an instant solidarity between us.

We all shook hands.

'So if you've been trying for five years, what's the

139

weirdest thing you've done to try and get pregnant?' I asked her.

'Well, I've done the usual things like yoga and acupuncture.'

My hand flew to my chest and I nodded vigorously, sensing she was a kindred spirit. 'Me, too!'

'Well, Gina makes me walk round in boxers that are ten sizes too big.' Karl put an arm around my shoulder.

'You, too?' Skinny Guy pulled a face. 'They're so uncomfortable!'

Karl and Skinny Guy nodded knowingly at each other.

Skinny Girl's head tilted to the side, thinking. 'The weirdest thing we did was a pagan fertility ritual at Stonehenge.'

'Wow!' I threw Karl a see-it's-not-just-me look.

'We nearly got arrested.' Skinny Guy raised an eyebrow. 'She made me prance around wearing a white sheet up there. It was so embarrassing.'

'Then there was another time we had sex at the Cerne Abbas Giant,' Skinny Girl said.

That's the fertility god I told you about in Dorset with the humongous willy, chalked out on a hillside.

I made a mental note to try both of her suggestions if the IVF didn't work out.

'What about you?' Skinny Girl asked me.

'Well, let me see…' I tapped my lips. 'I've feng shui-d the house.'

'Which actually meant completely wrecking the house and rewiring the TV.' Karl frowned at me.

'I didn't wreck the house!'

'You cut that really nice tree down in the front garden, and we had to take the original Twenties floorboards up in the lounge so we could run the TV wiring under them to the opposite side of the room.'

I waved a dismissive hand. 'I endured a nightmare yoga class that practically gave me a broken nose. I talk to the Universe. I wear crystals in my knickers. I've drunk weird concoctions that tasted like boiled up jock straps. I've spent a fortune on tarot text lines. Oh, yeah, and I did a fertility spell.' OK, now that I said all that it did sound slightly insane, but obviously I wasn't the only one on the baby trail doing weird stuff, which made me feel a whole lot better.

I glanced at Karl who didn't know about half of it. He shook his head at me silently.

'Really? I was thinking of doing a fertility spell,' Skinny Girl breathed with excitement. 'What did you have to do?

'Well…' I put my head conspiratorially towards hers as Skinny Guy and Karl started talking about football.

The Baby Trap

Karl was late for work in the morning and grumpy as he hunted for his keys, which wasn't a great start to the day, because my body was telling me that I was going to ovulate soon. I didn't want him in a bad mood because we'd need to have sex today, and again in two days to maximise any chance I had of fertilization. This would probably be the last month we had to conceive naturally before we started Herman's IVF treatment. One last shot at natural fertilization. I didn't think there was much chance, but the hope was still there, lurking under the surface.

'Where have you hidden them?' he said through a mouthful of toast.

'Hidden what?' I wandered into the converted garage where I did my beauty treatments and flicked on the overhead spotlights.

'You *know*.' He followed me in and gave me an accusing look, like I'd hidden them on purpose.

'If I knew, then I wouldn't be asking, would I?' I said.

'My keys. I can't find them.'

'They're probably in the usual place by the front door,' I muttered, scanning my appointment book. Did I really have eight Brazilian waxes booked in today? Now I'd spend all day looking up other people's lady gardens instead. How was that for messed up karma? Maybe Poppy was right about all that stuff. Before all this baby-making business started, I'd always loved my job. There was something fulfilling about being able to make people feel better and more confident about themselves. An upper lip wax here, eyebrow plucking there, a manicure. Now, I couldn't care less about it anymore. What good were perfect nails and hairless legs to me when I couldn't get pregnant?

'No, I looked there,' he huffed.

Why did I always have to sort everything out? No wonder I was stressed all the time. 'Maybe I accidentally mistook them for my hormone tablets and swallowed them,' I snapped, rolling my eyes at him.

'You haven't even started the hormone injections yet for the IVF. Are you getting moody already?'

'NO!' I rammed a tube of wax into the heater, my hormones standing to attention, ready to do battle, at the very mention of their name.

'Really?' He raised an eyebrow. 'You could've fooled me,' he growled, striding back into the kitchen.

Thank God men didn't have to go through fertility treatment. The whole population would be wiped out! But then it dawned on me that all this intolerable waiting to be a dad, and the worry about the upcoming IVF, must be hard on him, too. Men didn't like to show their feelings like women, did they? They didn't talk about such emotional things to their mates. I knew he was bottling it all up inside, trying to be strong for me. All the frustration, anger, and stress that I was going through, he must be feeling, too. There was no doubt that the IVF would be an intensive and invasive procedure. If the tables were turned, and I had to watch Karl go through everything that was involved, I think it would tear me to bits, so I was pretty sure he must be feeling the same. Even though I felt we were being a bit more proactive by starting IVF, now it seemed like the stakes had just got a whole lot higher, and the odds of winning were a whole lot lower.

I've now seen enough lady gardens to last a lifetime. Luckily one of my Brazilians wanted a Hollywood instead, which broke the monotony of the afternoon slightly, but managed to put me off my dinner. I couldn't get the thought of big lady gardens out of my head, especially since mine didn't seem to be flourishing at all. Still, at least it meant I'd have enough to pay for more gold-plated ovulation kits this month.

'Why don't we get a takeaway?' Karl's voice made me jump as I stared into the depths of the kitchen cupboards, trying to tempt my appetite back.

'Huh?' I swung round to face him.

'Curry or Chinese?' He rummaged around in the drawer where we kept the menus.

'Only if it's organic Chinese.' I grinned at him.

He peered at the menu. 'Yes, it says here organic sweet and sour chicken and organic spare ribs. They also do organic spring rolls.'

I flopped down on the chair at kitchen table and sighed. On the surface, it looked like I had everything I could want. A gorgeous husband who had a well-paid job. My own career as a beauty therapist. A lovely three-bedroomed house in a quiet part of town. We were both healthy. But one thing was missing, and it was something vital to me. I was giving the appearance of living my life, but my heart was only beating to become a mother. 'You *know* I've been sticking to this organic diet. People with fertility problems are more likely to get pregnant with no foreign or artificial products entering their bodies. I'm supposed to be putting only one-hundred percent natural ingredients into my body.'

'Ha! You don't say that when I'm sticking my product into you.' He smirked.

I giggled. He could still make me laugh, even after ten years together. Was that enough to get us through this? Sometimes I wasn't sure. I studied him for a few moments as my mind wandered, and a horrible thought popped into my head. If I had to make the choice between a baby and him, I would choose a baby. That sounds really horrible, doesn't it? It's nasty, irrational, and so desperately fucked-up, but that's how I felt at that moment. Don't get me wrong, I love him to bits, I was just...oh, I don't know. Bored, angry, depressed, anxious – take your pick. Exhausted, probably, by the rollercoaster of conflicting emotions that follow a cycle of treatment. Overwhelmingly angry at the world and the unfairness of everything. Worried and stressed about the IVF. Disappointed in the fact that I used to be happy, and now I could only focus on one thing.

'Gina?'

'Huh?' His voice brought me careening back to the present.

'I was just saying that one Chinese won't kill you. Everything in moderation: that's what I always say.' He paused. 'And you promised me that you wouldn't get so obsessed about all this baby stuff anymore.' He wrapped his arms around me and kissed my hair.

'I know, but it's easier said than done,' I mumbled into his shoulder.

It wasn't the same for him. He didn't get the same kind of feelings as me, which literally took over your brain and consumed it, like a maggot munching away.

'And I hate to tell you this,' I started, 'but it's that time of the month again when we have to do it. I've got my cervical mucus.'

I felt his shoulder stiffen beneath me.

And, to be honest, I probably felt the same as him. The last thing I felt like doing at that moment was having precision sex. Again. But needs must.

I lifted my head up and gazed into his dark brown eyes, trying to summon up some sort of arousal.

'Urgh! Do you have to keep going on about your mucus all the time? God, it makes me glad the no oral sex rule applies.' He pulled a disgusted face. 'Dining room, bedroom, kitchen table?' he asked in a monotone voice.

God, this is what we'd become. 'Well, the kitchen table's not great for keeping my legs in the air afterwards. It's a bit uncomfortable. Lounge floor?' I suggested, then took a step back and studied the hurt in his eyes. 'I'm sorry. I know this is difficult for you, too. All this pressure to perform.'

He pulled me back into his arms, stroking the back of my

145

head. 'Well, all this rushing about, having sex to order doesn't exactly inspire any fun in the romance department,' he sighed. 'And it's not just that. I hate seeing you go through this month after month, trying to keep your hopes up, only to see them dissolve when you don't get pregnant again. It makes me feel...I don't know...useless, I suppose. I can't make you happy anymore.'

I hugged him tighter. OK, I admit when I'm feeling at my lowest I did blame him sometimes for being unable to get pregnant. I know, I know, it wasn't his fault. His sperm was in tip-top condition. It's me who had the problem, so it was completely unfair of me to pass the buck onto him. I was the guilty one who couldn't give him what he wanted – children. I was the failure. And I knew deep down it wasn't his job to make me happy. Only I had the power to do that, but I was addicted to this obsession for a baby and that seemed to have totally whacked out my happy-ometer.

'You're caught in a trap,' he murmured, his voice sounding strangely far away.

'That sounds like an Elvis song,' I said, trying to make light of the situation.

'A baby trap. The only thing you can think about is getting pregnant, and I don't want to see you crumble apart again if the IVF doesn't work.' He squeezed me tighter so I could feel the beating of his heart. 'You're not living anymore. You're just existing.'

I sniffed as tears tingled in my eyes. 'I know,' I whispered into his neck.

'So you need to have a back-up plan.'

'What do you mean?'

'You need something else in your life to take your mind off it.'

'Hang on a sec, I thought you were the one who kept telling me to be positive all the time. Thinking about a back-up plan before we even begin the IVF is like saying you don't think it's going to work.'

'Not with you, it's not.'

146

'Huh?' I frowned. 'You're not making any sense.'

He took hold of my shoulders and looked deep into my eyes. 'I know you, Gina. Although you've been doing all these things to try and be positive that the fertility treatment will work, deep down you're worrying about it all the time. I just think that if you try and come up with some back-up plan for the future, it will get your mind off it. Don't they always say that as soon as people stop worrying about getting pregnant, it happens?

'Well...yes, I've heard that happens a lot,' I admitted reluctantly.

'And it's been proven that stress can negatively affect the outcome of IVF.' He paused. 'I know you're not going to be fulfilled doing your beauty business anymore. You need to think about doing something that's going to fill the hole if we can't have a baby so you can stop obsessing and chill out a bit.'

'Right. Like adoption, you mean, or surrogacy?'

He flopped down at the kitchen table, looking worn out. 'I can't do either of those things, Gina.' His gaze slid away from mine.

'What do you mean, you can't? Won't you even consider it?' I glared at him.

'I admire people who take on adoption, I really do. But it's not for everyone. I've been reading up on it a lot lately. You have to be prepared for all sorts of things. There aren't any babies to adopt in the UK, which means either taking on an older child, or trying to get a baby from another country.' He stood up and paced the floor. 'With an older child, most of them have been abandoned, abused, neglected, or institutionalised, and that can bring all sorts of emotional and psychological problems into it. And what about bonding issues? Attachment disorders? And some of the families still want access to the child, which would be incredibly difficult to cope with. The child would know we only adopted because we couldn't have our own baby, and I can only imagine how they'd feel about that.'

147

'But we would adopt because we want desperately to be parents,' I said.

'That isn't how they might see it. It's like marrying someone you don't love because the person you do love is taken.'

'So we can adopt a baby from abroad, then.'

'That can involve a whole set of other risks, and like surrogacy, we wouldn't know the medical history of the mother accurately. There's the possibility of the baby having foetal alcohol syndrome, brain damage, AIDS – so many things that you wouldn't find out about until the baby was older. A lot of the babies are from poor countries, where there's no proper pre or post natal care.' He pinched the bridge of his nose and sighed. 'What if it all went wrong and we blamed ourselves? Or, even worse, the child?' He shook his head. 'No, I'm just not cut out to adopt.'

Deep down I knew he was right. Even though I wanted desperately to be a parent, I didn't think I was cut out to adopt, either. I was terrified of ending up with a baby so psychologically scarred they wouldn't even speak, or one who had a terminal illness. I knew Karl was worried about the paternity issue with surrogacy and all those possible problems. And if I was honest, I didn't want Karl's sperm to fertilize another woman's eggs. I wanted them to have my genes to hand down to my baby.

The question is, what could possibly take the place of a baby for me? A cat? A dog? Hardly. A new career? Maybe. A fresh start somewhere else? God knows. Could I ever feel complete without a baby?

'But what can I do instead?' I whined, thinking maybe he had a point. Like Poppy said, it always seemed like when you really desperately wanted something in life, it never worked out. And yet, when you weren't that bothered, it seemed to happen easily. Maybe I could fool my brain into thinking I didn't want a baby and it would happen.

'That's something you have to figure out for yourself. It's not like we can't afford for you to do something different.

148

I'm earning enough to support both of us while you figure it out. But I want my wife back.' His voice took on an edge that I'd never heard before – a mixture of sadness and steely determination. 'Promise me you'll think about it.'

'I know!' I leapt back from him, blinking away the tears. 'How about I wear that black mini skirt you like with no knickers and my long, leather boots?' I rushed out of the room before he could answer, but as I disappeared up the stairs to get dressed I glanced back at him in the kitchen and saw him staring up at the ceiling, rubbing his forehead in an exhausted gesture. Were we one step closer to losing each other in all this?

Lying in bed that night my heart raced. I didn't know if it was anxiety about whether today was the day that Karl's sperm would finally fertilize my egg or not, or because I was thinking about what he'd said. No matter how hard I wracked my brains, I couldn't think of anything that would fulfil me anymore. Karl snoring like a wounded buffalo also put me off my train of thought.

I thought back to the conversation I'd had with Poppy earlier.

'I think Karl's right about getting something important in your life to take your mind off it. If you blank all thoughts about wanting a baby, I think it will happen. Just ask the Universe for guidance,' she said.

'Yes, I've been thinking about that, too, because Suzanne said something similar. So how do I go about that, exactly? I mean, do I just write it all down in a letter and address it to the Universe, Somewhere in Space, like I used to do with Santa's letters when I was a kid, or what?'

She chuckled. 'Not quite. Before you go to sleep tonight, imagine writing down your question on a piece of paper. Then imagine yourself folding it up and putting it into a small box.'

'Right, got it.' That sounded pretty easy. 'Then what?'

'Then imagine tying a balloon to the box and letting go of

it while you ask the Universe for guidance. Visualize the balloon floating away from you, and then switch off all thoughts about it.'

Ha! Easier said than done for Mrs Neurotic. 'OK.'

'The next morning the Universe will have your answer for you.'

'Great!' How simple was that?

'But it's not quite that simple,' she said.

Damn! I knew there had to be a catch.

'You have to learn to recognize the answer.'

Oh, for God's sake, why can't anything in life ever be simple? 'Er...what does that mean?'

'Well, the Universe may send you the answer in the form of a snippet of conversation you overhear, or a headline in a newspaper, or a piece of graffiti on a wall. There are hundreds of ways she might tune in to you. You just have to be aware of everything going on around you to pick it up.'

That sent me into panic mode. What if I missed it? What if she forgot to send me the answer or I misinterpreted it? It was perfectly possible to read a headline about something thinking it was for me, when maybe it was meant for someone else. Fuckety fuck! Why couldn't Zelda just have an email address?

'Oh, I've got to go,' Poppy said, distracting my thoughts. 'I've got my kundalini yoga class in half an hour.'

Her what? It sounded pretty rude to me. I have visions of naked yoga going on and...ew, a horrible thought appeared in my head.

'You should go to one. It's fantastic for unblocking your chakras and makes you feel fantastic.'

Not after the Taliban Torturer. There was no way in this lifetime I was going near a yoga class again. 'Yep, sounds good. One day I'll make sure I do.' I tried my most convincing voice. Bless her, she was only trying to help, but cunnilingus yoga? Come on!

****

So, as instructed, I was lying in bed with my eyes closed, taking deep breaths, silently repeating, my womb is a flower, my womb is a flower, my womb is a flower.

Karl did a little snore-grunt and turned over. I hoped I wasn't saying it out loud. He would get me sectioned soon.

OK, next, on to the letter…

I took an extra long deep breath and imagined writing on a pink piece of paper. Then I scrapped it and used a white piece. What if Zelda hated the colour pink and jinxed me? White couldn't offend anyone, could it? No.

So, here we go again.

White piece of paper. Check!

Question scrawled on it:

Zelda, I know you don't know me, but I was wondering if you could help enlighten me as to my purpose in life if I can't get pregnant. Can you please send me a message to tell me how I can fill this colossal hole in my heart and head.

P.S. Could you also make it easy to spot your answer, please?

Thanks so much!

Gina xxx

P.P.S. Do you have an email address?

Here goes!

I folded the paper into the box, tied a balloon to it, and let it go, imagining it floating into the starlit night. Up, up, and away, until it was just a speck in the distance.

One more deep breath for luck, then I turned over and banished it from my mind.

A Sign?

Snoring, grunting and whinnying from Karl did not abate all night. I had weird dreams that Zelda was a unicorn and sent me a message while I was in the supermarket. The only problem was that the message was on a packet of frozen sausages that said, "Buy One Get One Free." What the hell was that supposed to mean? Was that her answer, or was it just a stupid dream? Now I'm more confused than ever.

I've been trying to tune in to Zelda to try and find her answer for me. Somehow, I've got a feeling this is going to be a very long day. OK, it started with breakfast TV. I thought maybe there would be a sign for me there because I watch it all the time. I ate my porridge (organic, of course) with a sprinkle of raisins (yuck, I hate them, but they're healthy) and Manuka honey (good for all sorts, apparently), and concentrated on the screen like never before. What was I looking for, though? I didn't have a clue. There was an interview with a pop star who was becoming an ambassador for an animal charity, the weatherman talking about a hurricane in the US, and an advert in the break for Nike – the slogan was "Just Do It."

What did it all mean? Something or nothing? Was I meant to volunteer to help out at disaster zones in the world? While it was a very noble cause, and I admired anyone who did that kind of work, I didn't think Karl would be too impressed about that. I could just imagine the conversation...

'Hi, darling, I'm just running off to Miami to do a spot of rebuilding work after the hurricane.'

'What? You can't even put a nail in the wall? And the last time you tried to use a drill we needed to have the whole wall re-plastered.'

Hmmm…you see my dilemma?

Or how about working with animals? I loved animals. The only trouble was that Karl had a fur allergy, so how could I be around cats and dogs and fluffy bunnies all day without it transferring onto my clothes?

No, that couldn't be it.

The Nike message was crystal clear. *Just Do It*. But what the hell was I supposed to be doing?

Then the paper arrived! Yay! Maybe there was something from Zelda in there. The headlines on the first page read, "Local Councillor having an affair with parishioner!"

Omigod! Was that Zelda's answer? I was supposed to have an affair? And if so, why? An affair? Nope. That couldn't be it.

Maybe I was supposed to be a local councillor. Help out the community and all that. That was definitely a possibility.

Oh, this is ridiculous!

I ended up slinging the paper in the bin before I could jump to any more stupid conclusions.

After back-to-back clients all day, I felt claustrophobic in the house. A walk in the fresh air would do me good. Plus, I couldn't shake the thought that maybe there was something in this message business, and what if Zelda was sending the messages somewhere outside and not inside?

I bundled myself up in my thick wool coat, wrapped a soft pink scarf around my neck, and took a deep breath as I pulled the door open.

My womb is a flower (I was still repeating that, just in case).

Thoughts rambled about in my head as I walked off down the street, peeking in the windows of the detached houses. At least the sun was shining, doing its best to bite into the bitter chill of the afternoon.

I heard children shrieking behind the bay windows of one house and caught a glimpse of a couple of toddlers hitting each other over the head with blow-up toys. I swallowed down a lump in my throat and tried to ignore a tightness spreading across my chest.

Don't cry, Gina. Don't do it!

I tore my gaze away from their window and forced myself to look ahead, just in time to see a young mother pushing a pram towards me.

Bitch! It's sooooo not fair! Don't I deserve children, too?

She smiled at me as she passed but I couldn't summon even a crinkle in the corners of my lips. I blinked hard to try and stop my vision from blurring with salty tears and stumbled on the pavement in my high-heel boots.

Stop it, Gina. Focus. Pull yourself together and look for the message!

I brushed away the tears, willing myself to think about anything except babies. Mrs Omeroyd's pig's trotters managed to get my train of thought moving in the right direction as I strolled towards the park at the end of the road.

No, don't go in there! Too many children playing that you won't want to see. Don't torture yourself.

I strolled past, turning my head in the opposite direction so I wasn't tempted to look, and immediately spied an advert for a watch on the bus stop. "You'll never run out of time with a Timex."

Could that be it? Did it mean I'd get pregnant soon? Was Zelda telling me not to give up? That there was plenty of time?

As I walked down the high street, the wind suddenly whipped up to tornado level and blew me towards a shop. It was so powerful that I was unable to stop myself getting swept along. And then the next second, I'd landed in front of a travel agent, and the wind had completely disappeared, as if I'd just imagined the whole thing.

I glanced around me to see if anyone else had noticed the sudden bizarre wind, but the high street had morphed into a ghost town and no one was around.

I thought about what Poppy and Suzanne had said about

looking for signs from the Universe. Could this be what Zelda was trying to tell me? Call me crazy (and I'm sure you have. Many times!), but somehow I just knew it was.

My heart broke into a tap-dancing beat and a surge of adrenaline shot through me as I stood, staring at the poster in the travel agent's window.

Discover Australia.

I scanned the poster, devouring it with my eyes.

There were pictures of golden beaches; turquoise waters with colourful fish that made you want to dive in, right there and then. A rock in the middle of the outback with the sun setting behind it, giving it an ethereal glow. Fireworks going off at a crowded Sydney Harbour Bridge.

It all looked so inviting.

Yep, I was sure this was meant for me.

I went inside, the bell above the door jangling to announce my arrival.

A young girl looked up from her desk. 'Hi. Can I help you?'

'I'd like some brochures on Australia, please,' I announced.

She stood up and walked to the brochure rack. 'Well, this one is good for package holidays. This is one from the Australian Tourist Board for backpacking holidays and longer stays travelling around the country.' She handed them to me. 'And here are a few more.'

The brochures felt both heavy and magically hot in my hands.

'That should keep you busy for a while.' She smiled.

I hugged them to my chest as I retraced my journey back to the house with a new bounce in my step.

As soon as I got through the door I flung my coat haphazardly on the coat rack, kicked off my boots, and rushed to the phone in the kitchen to call Poppy.

'I think it was a sign,' I said after I'd told her what had happened.

'To go on holiday to Australia?' Poppy asked.

'No. I don't think just for a holiday. We could go and travel around, for a year, maybe. Discover a whole new country. Get our life back again and stop obsessing about babies. Have time for us for a change,' I said breathlessly, flicking through the brochure, which was packed with sunny skies, beautiful countryside, and amazing open spaces. 'I always wanted to take a year out and backpack around Oz when I was a teenager, but I never got around to it. And then I got tied down to a job and a mortgage, and eventually I met Karl. It's like Zel...I mean, the Universe is trying to rekindle that idea I had when I was younger.'

'Well, yes, why not?' She laughed. 'The Universe works in mysterious ways.'

'It could be perfect. Drive around in one of those campervans they hire out, stopping wherever the mood takes us. No plans, just going with the flow.' My mind was racing as I thought about it. 'We could rent our house out to pay for it.'

'But what about Karl's job?'

Hmmm. I hadn't thought about that. Oh, well, it was early days, but this was at least a starting point. 'I don't know. I haven't even discussed it with Karl yet. I need to think about it a bit more.'

'Erm...well, I've got some news, too,' Poppy said, her voice quivering with excitement. 'I'm finally pregnant!' she breathed hard down the phone. 'The IVF worked!'

Bitch, was my first thought, closely followed by cow and trout. It was so unfair. Why could Poppy get pregnant and I couldn't? Did she deserve it more than me? And if so, who decided that? Then an overwhelming feeling of guilt swept over me. I was a horrible person for even thinking that. Poppy had been trying for four years, and it was her third round of IVF.

'I'm so happy for you.' I masked my jealousy with a gushing voice, even though the empty, hollow feeling in my stomach was growing by the second.

'I...I didn't know whether to tell you or not. I know how

156

upsetting it is to hear about when someone else falls pregnant. It's OK to hate me' She chuckled. 'Well, not for long! But...I'm still going to be here to talk to you about everything, and support you through the bad times.'

'No...I...' OK, she was right. I did hate her at that moment, but it wasn't her fault. Poppy had been such a good friend to me, and she deserved to be happy. I was turning into the nasty, jealous kind of person that I despised, but I felt powerless to stop it. 'I really hope everything goes OK.' I felt the tears trickling down my cheeks and my throat constricting. All I wanted to do was get off the phone. 'I've got to go now. I'll phone you tomorrow,' I croaked.

I kicked the wooden door to the kitchen after I'd hung up.

Ouch!

I rubbed at my foot and hopped to the kitchen table, slumping forward with my head in my arms as salty tears soaked my face.

Why couldn't it be me?

'Gina,' Karl called out from the hallway as he slammed the front door. 'God, I've had such a crap day at the office.'

I heard him putting his briefcase down and wandering into the kitchen where I was still in the same position. Sod dinner. I couldn't even think about that now. Karl could get the bloody Chinese takeaway he'd been lusting after. Hell, maybe I'd ignore this stupid organic diet and have one, too. It wasn't like it seemed to be doing any good, was it?

'These sales figures they keep trying to get me to meet are more and more ridiculous every day. I'm under so much pressure to...' he trailed off as I lifted my head and gave him a weak smile.

He stood there staring at me. 'What's up?'

That started a fresh round of waterworks as I told him through sniffs and gulps of air about Poppy.

'Ah.' He flopped down next to me, putting his arm around me, gently stroking my shoulder. 'Sorry.'

Sorry? Was that it? It was such a little word, and it

sounded so inconsequential under the circumstances. Sorry Poppy is going to have a precious, miracle baby, and not you. Sorry you're so useless you can't even do something simple that millions of women in the world manage to do with no problems. Sorry it's not your time yet. Honestly, sometimes I thought he just wasn't interested in a baby. Sorry?

Hot flames of anger engulfed me. 'Is that all you can say, sorry? You've been saying sorry for nearly two years!'

He removed his arm, stood up, and paced the black tiles on the kitchen floor. 'Exactly,' he said, smooth and controlled. 'I don't know what to say anymore. What do you want me to say?'

I threw my hands up in an impatient gesture. 'I don't know!'

He stared around the kitchen. 'Are we having dinner? I'm starving. I missed lunch to have an important meeting.'

I jumped off the chair. 'FUCK DINNER!' I stormed off upstairs and slammed the bedroom door.

'Oh, now I've got to fuck the dinner, too!' he yelled up at me.

I threw myself on the bed, trying to practise some deep breathing.

My womb is a flower, my womb is a flower. My womb is a fucking useless waste of space!

Downstairs, Karl banged around in the kitchen cupboards and I heard the phone ring and muffled voices. Everything going on around me as normal, except here I was, teetering on the edge of a ravine of despair. One little slip and I'd tip over the edge to God knows where.

Come on, Gina. Keep it together. Get a grip. It's not Karl's fault. It's not your fault.

Yeah, right! It is my fault.

Calm down. The IVF will work.

****

158

'Gina.' Karl hovered in the bedroom doorway a few hours later, the light from the hallway behind spilling into the darkened room. 'Amelia's on the phone. Do you want to talk to her?'

I nodded and swung my legs off the bed, grabbing the phone on the table next to me. 'Hi,' I whispered as the door clicked shut behind him again.

'Hey! How are you? You sound down, what's happened?'

I took a deep breath. 'Nothing.' My friends were getting sick of me going on about babies all the time. Karl was getting sick of me going on about it. Even I was getting sick of me. And unless someone was going through the same thing, they just didn't get the excruciating pain of being infertile. It's the equivalent of losing all your children if you were lucky enough to have them in the first place. You grieve every single day for something that you've never even had yet. I picked up the picture of Mum next to my bed and stared at it. She would've understood. I had my friends and Karl but I felt cut off and lonely. Only Poppy and the girls on the fertility forum completely understood what it was like.

I forced my voice to sound brighter and put on my happy face. 'Nothing. I'm OK.'

'Hmm,' she said, not sounding convinced. 'You sound pissed off.'

'Oh, we've just had a bit of a row. You know, the usual.'

'I see. Well, I'm your saviour then. Do you fancy going out for a drink on Friday night? Kick off your shoes, have a boogie and a laugh. It might help to take your mind off things,' she said.

That sounded so tempting, but gone were the days when I could sink a couple of bottles of wine with my friends. 'I'd love to, but I might be tempted to drink lots of wine and get pissed, and I need to stay off the booze still if I want to be in tip-top shape for the IVF. Why don't you come round here instead?'

'Sounds like a plan!' she said, then paused for a beat. 'Is it

OK if Kerry comes, too? She thinks you've been avoiding her since she started showing.'

I sighed, feeling like the most horrible friend in the whole world. 'I have kind of been avoiding her. It's just so difficult to see her now she's getting bigger.'

'She knows it's not easy for you, and she feels really bad.'

I could've kicked myself. I was so wrapped up in my own life that I hadn't even stopped to think about how Kerry was feeling at being pushed away by me. 'Yes, I'll make sure I invite her.'

'Good. She'll be really pleased to see you.'

'Anyway, how are you and Dan?'

'Oh, we're good, now he's got his shed! He's building a train set in there for his sister's oldest boy. Actually, I think he's really building it for himself. His nephew is just an excuse. They never grow up, do they? Still, it means I can watch what I want to on TV and there's no fight over the remote. I've got it all figured out.' She laughed.

I envied the sound of her laid-back laughter. I wished I had it all figured out. 'Men and their sheds.'

'Yep. OK, I'll see you about eight on Friday?'

'Looking forward to it,' I said. And I was. Amelia was always happy and bubbly, just like I used to be. Nothing ever seemed to faze her. I wanted some of her positive vibes to rub off on me.

I hung up and wandered downstairs, needing to clear the air with Karl. I hated sleeping on an argument. It always made things ten times worse. I could never get to sleep, just tossing and turning with things running through my head, and I needed a calm womb.

The TV was on quietly in the lounge and Karl was flopped out on our black, leather sofa, tuned in to *Top Gear*. Amelia was right. Give a man a car or a shed and he'd be happy.

I stood over him, taking his hand in mind. 'I'm sorry I flew off the handle.'

He took my hand and pulled me on top of him, holding me tight.

'It's just–'

'I know,' he cut me off, squeezing me close so his heartbeat resounded in my chest. 'Believe me, I know. Are you going out with Amelia?'

'No.'

'It'll do you good. You need to go out, have a change of scenery.'

I tipped my face towards him and kissed his soft lips, suddenly so grateful to have him. It wasn't his fault things had worked out the way they had. 'Because if I do, I'll be tempted to have too much to drink, and you know that might mess up my body.'

'Well, maybe that's exactly what you need.' He eyed me. 'You need to get out and have some fun. Relax for a change and stop thinking about babies for five minutes.'

'No, Amelia and Kerry are coming here for a girlie night in instead.'

'I'll pop over and drag Dan and Mark to the pub when she gets here, then. Give you girls some peace.'

'OK. But please don't have too much to drink. Alcohol can affect the quality of your sperm,' I said, painfully aware that I was sounding like a stuck record.

'Mmm, don't I know it!'

Nurse Awful

We arrived for our first appointment at the hospital half an hour early. As we took a seat in the waiting room, I couldn't believe the amount of women sitting there who were pregnant. Didn't they have a separate waiting room for them? Talk about rub your nose in it!

I sat down next to Karl and grabbed a magazine, burying my head in it so I wouldn't have to look at them. I was just getting a headache and eyestrain when a Scottish nurse called Claire finally called for us.

I threw the magazine down on the table and stared at my feet as we followed her to the doctor's office.

'I'm Dr Jansen.' A man with bushy black hair and half-moon glasses stood and reached his hand out with a welcoming smile. He didn't look like Herman Munster, which was a relief. Not a weird-shaped head or neck bolt in sight. He was spick and span from top to toe in a pin-striped suit and tie and a white doctor's coat, and looked like someone who would iron their boxer shorts.

'Hi.' I nervously shook his hand.

He gave me a firm handshake in return. That was good, wasn't it? Didn't a firm handshake mean he was confident? Good at his job? Hopefully.

'Nice to meet you,' Karl said as we sat down.

'First, I need to take your medical history.' Dr Jansen clicked the top of his biro and began writing notes as we explained our history in detail. He asked us various questions and took more notes.

162

'We need to take some more tests from you at this stage,' he said, ticking them off on his fingers. 'Gina, we need to do a transvaginal scan on you. Karl, we need you to do another sperm test, and we need to take various blood tests from both of you. Just to get an idea of how things stand at the moment. If the tests come back normal, then we can start your IVF treatment at the beginning of your next cycle.'

Hurrah! Bring it on!

After my scan, which appeared to be perfectly OK (thank God!), Claire took us off to the pathology department to wait for our blood tests.

With those completed, all that was left was Karl's sperm sample.

'I'm afraid we're a bit busy today and we've run out of private cubicles at the moment,' a scary-looking nurse said. She was so short and stocky, she reminded me of a munchkin. She looked like she'd been at the hormone treatments herself, complete with a big Adam's apple and a thick spattering of upper-lip hair. I was dying to get my wax out and whip if

t off for her. Any minute now I expected her to break into a rendition of "Follow the Yellow Brick Road."

She led us into a corridor that had doors with "occupied" on them. 'The only room available is the cleaner's storage cupboard,' she grunted.

Karl looked at me in horror, then back at the nurse.

'Er...can we wait for a private cubicle to become free?' Karl asked, looking uncomfortable at the thought of doing it in a cupboard.

She made a huge point of sighing and glancing at her watch. 'It's half past five now and the clinic will be closing soon. You can always come back tomorrow. Or if you live within a couple of hours travelling time I can give you a sample cup to bring back.'

Karl sighed, glancing at me. 'I've got meetings all day tomorrow. I'll have to leave home about 6 a.m. as it is.' He paused for a moment. 'No, it's OK. We can use the cleaner's

163

cupboard.'

'Would you like some magazines?' She asked with a smirk, as if she were enjoying this.

Ew. I dreaded to think what kind of state they were in. By the look on Karl's face, he was thinking the same thing.

'No, thanks,' Karl said. 'I'm sure I'll be able to manage.'

'Right you are, then.' Nurse Awful stopped in front of a door marked "Cleaners" and opened it, turning the light on. 'Your suite awaits you.' She grinned.

Karl and I stepped in and she closed the door.

'Great. I've got to have a wank in a broom cupboard. And on top of that, I'm paying three grand for the privilege. And where's the lock?' Karl stared at the door, eyes wide. 'There's no lock. What if someone barges in?'

I snorted. 'No one's going to barge in.'

'Oh, yeah, I thought that at the hotel and Clive barged in.'

We glanced around the tiny cupboard for something to shove in front of the door. Mops, wide brooms, containers of disinfectant, a couple of nurses' uniforms hanging up, a plastic chair.

'There.' I pointed to the chair. 'Shove it under the handle of the door.'

Karl scraped it across the floor and positioned it carefully. Checking and re-checking the handle to see if someone could push it open. When he was satisfied, he looked around the grey cupboard, which was lit by a dim bulb.

'Doesn't exactly inspire me to get in the mood,' he grumbled, looking at the mops. 'There's nowhere to sit because we've shoved that chair under the door, and there's nowhere to lie down.'

'What's wrong with doing it standing up?' I asked, stepping close to him.

I closed my eyes and kissed him, stroking my hand up and down his back. After a little while, he seemed to relax a bit so I moved my hands to his crotch, massaging him gently through the fabric of his jeans. I felt him stiffen underneath me and glanced up at him, eyebrow raised. 'How about now? Are you in the mood?'

'Mmmm,' he mumbled. 'That's pretty good.'

I undid the zip and slid my hand in between his jeans and baggy boxers just as I heard a pair of high heels clacking along the tiled flooring in the corridor outside, getting louder and louder.

Karl froze, pushing my hand away. 'Someone's coming.'

We both turned to look at the door, expecting someone to burst in, but the heels carried on past and disappeared into the distance.

'That's probably a patient or doctor wearing heels,' I said. 'A cleaner isn't going to be wearing stilettos.' I turned back to him. 'Now, where were we?' I resumed stroking a now very soft willy.

After about five more minutes, he was getting back into the swing of things when we heard a doctor with a really loud voice talking to a patient in the room next door. 'So, the nurse was just telling me you think that the hormone injections are causing your diarrhoea,' he said.

'Yes, Doctor. It only started since I've been on them,' the patient said.

'And what colour is the diarrhoea?' the doctor said.

'Great!' Karl threw his hands in the air. 'I'm trying to get turned on and someone's talking about their toilet habits!'

After a few minutes, and no more bodily fluid references, I resumed crotch duty.

'Oh, this isn't working!' Karl exhaled a frustrated breath. 'It's all right for women, you can just close your eyes and think about Brad Pitt and get horny. Men need visual stimulation.' He looked around the cupboard with narrowed eyes.

'How about we spice things up a bit and make it more visual?' I glanced at the nurses' outfits and hastily pulled one of them over the broom, giggling. 'What do you think? Is she turning you on?' I held it out, grinning, trying to bring some humour into the situation to get him to relax. 'Is she visual enough for you? If you look at her from the right

165

angle she looks a bit like Angelina Jolie, doesn't she?'

Karl glared at me.

'What? You're always going on about how much you fancy her!'

More glaring. On a scale of one to ten glaring this was triple digits.

I put my hand up. 'OK, OK, *I'll* put the uniform on.' And just as I said that, there was a knock at the door.

'Sorry to disturb you, but I need to get the broom,' a voice said from the other side of the door.

In Karl's rush to do up his zip in case she walked in, he caught his wedding tackle in it. 'Agh!' He winced, screwing his eyes shut, head turned up to the ceiling, letting out a silent scream.

'Just a minute!' I said, removing the chair and opening the door a smidgen so I could slide out the broom, which was now wearing the nurse's outfit.

A young girl with a pierced nose and spiky hair raised her eyebrows at me. 'Whatever floats your boat.' She chuckled as I slammed the door shut and replaced the chair.

Karl carried on glaring, but this time at the door. 'For fuck's sake,' he whispered. 'This is ridiculous!'

'Well, *I'll* just put on the nurse outfit, then.' I stripped off, doing a slinky impression of a striptease and acting as seductive as you can when you're stuck in a broom cupboard, trying to turn your husband on.

'That's more like it.' Karl allowed himself a slight grin as I pulled on the nurse outfit.

'I'm Nurse Angelina and I need your sperm,' I said in a husky voice, beckoning him towards me as I licked my lips.

Letting Go

I was looking forward to my next appointment with Suzanne. I'd been trying really hard to do what she said, to trust that everything would work out and then forget about it, but it was like telling a crack addict that they couldn't think about getting their fix anymore. Not that I'd ever smoked crack, you understand, (although there was one time in college when I smoked a joint) but it just seemed like an impossible task.

'How have things been?' Suzanne gave me a warm hug as she greeted me at the door.

'I've been feeling a lot calmer since our session.' Then I paused. 'Well, some of the time,' I added with a laugh. 'I've turned into an uptight, impatient stress-head since we started trying for a baby.'

'It's understandable, but you need to keep working on it. Come on, let's go to the treatment room.'

'I've been avoiding one of my friends who's pregnant and I feel so guilty about it. It's not that I'm not happy for her, I really am. It's just so painful to see other people with big baby bumps. And another friend I met online through the fertility website is also pregnant now. It just feels like it's happening for everyone except me.' I sat down on the treatment couch.

She nodded. 'Jealousy is a normal emotion, but again, it's a negative energy that will affect your chakras.' She paused for a moment. 'You need to try and turn all negatives into positives, and pretty soon you'll find you're happier and it actually enhances your life.'

'But how can I do that?'

167

'The way you should look at it is that if it's possible for someone else to get pregnant, then it's possible for you to, as well. Success and happiness is infinite. Just because someone else has succeeded doesn't mean you won't.' She sat next to me, taking my cold hands in her warm ones. 'When someone is doing well in life, or has achieved what they want, you should be genuinely happy for them. The happier you are for them, the more those things will come around to you. It's all about good karma.'

I took all this in, jotting down everything in my memory bank so I could think about it later.

'So instead of being jealous of your friends, congratulate them, and genuinely mean it. Be happy for them. Don't feel miserable about things or harbour resentments. Have confidence and trust that everything in the Universe is connected and then you are lighter and free to enjoy your journey in life instead of just focusing on your end goal or destination and missing out on the here and now.'

She was right. Everything she said always made sense. I would ring Kerry when I got home and apologize to her for keeping my distance.

'Did you do the visualization exercise I told you about last time, where you focus on achieving your pregnancy and then let it go?'

'No.' I gave her a sheepish grin. 'I promise I will. But I have been trying to think about what I'm going to do with my life if I can't get pregnant so it stops me obsessing so much about the IVF. I'm turning into someone I don't recognize with the stress and hormones flying around all over the place. I mean, when I look in the mirror it's still me staring back, but it's not really *me,* if you know what I mean.' I glanced up at the ceiling and sighed. 'But at the same time, I know I can't go back to the old me I was before all this started because that would be impossible. Now there's something in me that's missing, so I need to do something drastic to either fill the gap or focus on instead.' I turned back to her and smiled. 'And I did actually ask Zel…I

168

mean, the Universe for some guidance.' I chuckled. If Karl could hear me now he'd think I was bonkers.

'Really, that's the second step to the visualization process I was talking about. After you take the first step, the next is to get on with your life. Look for guidance or intuition in what you're supposed to be doing. It's not an either/or situation. The Universe, or God, or whoever you want to believe in, doesn't say, "OK, you can't be mother so that's it, your life is over." It goes back to the trust thing: trusting that it will happen, then forgetting about it and getting on with your life. Then something fulfilling or some opportunity will come to you.'

I was so going to do that exercise when I got home.

'And all this experience you've been going through is bound to have an effect on your self-esteem and self-confidence,' she went on. 'You need to love yourself and be happy with yourself before you can love others fully and get happiness from your life again.'

All this emotional talk brought more tears to my eyes, and I wiped them away with the heel of my hand.

'Just take everything one step at a time.' She gave my hands a quick squeeze and let go of them. 'Now lie back and relax, and I'll start the treatment.'

The first thing I did when I got back to the house was call Kerry and apologize for avoiding her. She was great about it. She understood completely, and I did feel my mood lighten because of it.

Jealousy is out. Happiness is in. Woo hoo!

Then I went upstairs and lay on the bed, closing my eyes, thinking about everything that Suzanne had said.

I breathed deeply for a while before summoning up an image in my head of my baby. It was a girl, and I actually called her Zelda (maybe I'd get extra Brownie points for that!). She was beautiful. She had Karl's hair and my almond-shaped eyes. Her ears were small and cute, and she had a button nose that was so precious. I held her in my arms and rubbed my nose against hers, sniffing her gorgeous baby smell. She giggled back at me with happiness.

I thought about my motives for wanting her in my life. I wanted to teach her things so she would grow up to be a good person. I wanted to cherish her and nourish her. I wanted to appreciate the miracle of her. I wanted to enjoy her – see her flourish into a blossoming woman. I wanted to love her unconditionally and have fun with her. I thought about how she would enhance my life. She would make it fuller, richer. Yes, there would be times when she'd be a complete pain in the arse, but she would bring fun and enjoyment and depth to us that couldn't be gained by any other thing in life.

I pictured everything in my mind for half an hour, but I knew I'd have to let it go. Banish it from my thoughts completely, like Suzanne had said, and trust Zelda to bring it to me.

I took a deep breath and opened my eyes. No more vision.

Now I'd spend time concentrating on my life.

Karl and Britney

Karl arrived home minus his tie and reeking of perfume, so the night didn't start off too well. This wasn't the first time! Either he was going through a midlife crisis and stealing my *Fantasy* by Britney Spears or he was having an affair.

Agh! Maybe that was it. Maybe he *was* having an affair. Had I been pushing him away so much, lost in my own crisis, that I hadn't noticed the warning signs?

I got a waft of Britney as he sauntered into the room, looking slightly dishevelled. I stirred the tomato, garlic, and roasted pepper sauce (all organic, of course) and glared at him.

'What have I done now?' He undid his first two shirt buttons and poured himself a glass of non-alcoholic wine.

'Are you having an affair with Britney Spears, or couldn't you find your aftershave this morning?' I stopped mid-stir and scrutinized his face for signs of devious behaviour. But what did devious behaviour look like?

Wait a sec, did he just glance shiftily at his briefcase? What did that mean?

Omigod, even worse thought! Maybe this was the sign from Zelda. After all, there'd been the headlines on the newspaper about the councillor having an affair. What if the Australia poster wasn't a sign from her at all? What if she was really trying to tell us to split up? Get a divorce? Tell us our relationship wasn't working anymore? We'd been under so much stress for nearly two years with all this baby business, it was bound to put pressure on us. And, let's face it, I hadn't exactly been fun to be around lately. I thought back to how we'd met ten years ago. Amelia, Kerry, and I

171

had been in a nightclub, having a photo competition of who could have the most photos take with the most guys. I won. Then we'd got bored of that game (which we thought was hilarious at the time), and spied an empty dancer's pole next to the bar. Of course, I had to have a go. But strangely, two bottles of wine and swinging around a pole at high velocity didn't seem to mix, and I lost my grip, falling off and landing slap bang on top of Karl, who was standing at the bar trying to order a pint of beer. That was the woman Karl fell in love with – the slightly crazy, lively, anything-for-a-laugh girl – until the past few years had turned me into a dull, lifeless party-pooper who didn't know how to have a good time anymore. Could I really blame him if he wanted to have an affair?

Fuck! A cold sliver of fear danced up my spine.

His intense brown eyes gazed back at me. 'Sometimes I don't have clue what you're talking about.' He sipped his wine, a puzzled look sweeping over his face.

'Well that makes two of us, then. But that's not the point.'

'So what is?'

I grated some parmesan vigorously. Too vigorously, actually, and the whole block exploded in a cheesy, lumpy heap in the dish. 'You coming home stinking of perfume. *That's the point.*'

He pulled his collar out and sniffed at it like a dog. 'I can't smell anything except garlic.'

I threw him a suspicious look. 'Why do you smell like the perfume counter at Boots, then?' I slopped the pasta into some bowls, spooned the sauce on top, and slammed them on the kitchen table.

He sipped his wine, looking sheepish. There was definitely something going on.

Or was I just being oversensitive?

'For fuck's sake, Gina! Stop being so paranoid about everything.' He plonked himself down at the table, avoiding my gaze. Instead, he directed his attention to the pasta that he hated.

'I'm not being paranoid. You've been acting weird for ages.'

'Well, that makes two of us, then.' He exhaled a heavy sigh. 'It's your birthday soon, isn't it?'

'Yes,' I muttered slowly, hoping this was going to be a good explanation, otherwise I could see the entire dinner going over his head.

'So, if you must know, I went to John Lewis on the way home and was trying out some tester perfumes for a present. If you don't believe me, have a look in my briefcase, but you'll ruin the surprise.' He glanced up.

I smiled with relief. How stupid of me to think he was having an affair. I kicked myself under the table as I sat down. Of course he wouldn't do that. He loved me.

He peered at his dinner, his lip curling up in disgust. 'Urgh. Are we eating worms again?' He poked his fork in and pulled out some pasta, staring at it like it was going to rear up and bite him on the nose.

'It's good for you. Eat it.' I took a mouthful and grimaced. What I wouldn't do for a very un-organic pizza or burger and chips. Why did the good stuff always taste horrible?

After Karl disappeared to the pub to "have a normal conversation with my friends, rather than talking to a non-normal, hormonal woman," Amelia and Kerry arrived bearing gifts of wine and Galaxy bars. Once again, I had to think of my healthy diet and deprive myself of scrummy chocolate and stick to one glass of non-alcoholic elderflower wine. Oh, OK, maybe two. Whoopee!

Hugs all round, and an extra special one for Kerry.

'Oh, you've got so big!' I said.

Feel genuine happiness. It will come back to you.

I stepped back to check out her bump. Then I reached my hand out and touched it.

Amelia watched me with a worried look. She probably thought I was about to rip the baby out of Kerry's stomach there and then and run off with it.

173

'It's OK, guys! I'm OK,' I said. 'I've been seeing this fantastic woman who's helping me look at things differently.'

'Only two weeks to go!' Kerry said with a beaming smile, rubbing her stomach.

Don't punch her. Be happy for her.

I hugged her again. 'You're so lucky,' I said, without a trace of jealousy. OK, maybe a teeny tiny bit, but hey, I was only human! 'How's Mark? Is he meeting Dan and Karl down the pub?'

'No.' Kerry's eyes sparkled with love. 'He's putting the finishing touches to the nursery. We're doing it in lavender and butterscotch. Oh, it's so gorgeous!'

'How is everything between you?' Amelia asked her.

She waved a hand. 'Fantastic! Great! It's amazing. We click on every level, and he's been so kind and supportive. I can't wait to marry this one!'

'I'm not talking to you.' I pointed a finger at Amelia as I uncorked her wine and poured out a big glass, drooling as I looked at it. 'How can you bring wine and chocolate round and I can't even have any.'

Amelia gave me a sheepish grin. 'Sorry.' But she didn't seem that sorry as she took a sip and said, 'Oh, that is sooooooo good!'

'Oooh, you bitch!' I grinned.

Kerry took the glass off her and sniffed it. 'Yep, I miss this, too. Maybe we should confiscate it.' She looked at me and held the glass high in the air so Amelia couldn't reach it.

'Hey! Stop ganging up on me.' Amelia swung her arm through the air, trying to reach it.

'You wouldn't fight with a pregnant woman, would you?' Kerry faked a stern look.

Amelia rolled her eyes. 'I can tell this is going to be a long night.'

We made our way into the lounge and sat on the sofas – well, Kerry waddled and then spent five minutes easing herself up and down, trying to get comfortable.

'So how's the treatment going? Tell us all about it.' Amelia gushed, curling her legs underneath her.

'Hang on, I'll tell you in a minute. First you have to do me a favour and look in Karl's briefcase.' I fiddled with the locks on it and then broke my fingernail. 'Shit.' I peered at my nail.

'Why?' She half-laughed, half-frowned at me.

The locks pinged open. 'Here.' I passed the case to her. 'I think he might be having an affair. I need you to look inside and tell me if there's a bottle of perfume inside.'

She rested her glass on the floor. 'He is *not* having an affair.' She laughed. 'Have you gone mad? He'd never do that to you.'

'Of course he wouldn't,' Kerry agreed.

I gave them a knowing look and folded my arms across my chest. 'Go on. Have a look.' I nodded my head towards it impatiently.

Amelia sighed and opened it. 'There's a—'

I put my hand up to stop her.

'What?' she laughed. 'You said you wanted to know what's in it!'

'Just tell me if there's a bottle of perfume in there. But don't tell me what it is if there is one,' I said, trying to avoid peeking inside myself.

Amelia shook her head and snorted. 'Yes,' she said.

'Yes, what?' I said, a bad, bubbling sensation creeping from my stomach up to my chest. 'Yes, there is perfume in there, or yes, you think he's having an affair?'

'Yes, there is perfume in there.' She closed it firmly and put it back on the floor.

I nodded thoughtfully. 'Hmm.' So he was telling the truth. 'What sort is it?' I raised an eyebrow.

'Not telling.' Amelia giggled. 'You said you didn't want to know. And anyway, I'm sure it's supposed to be a surprise. Why do you think he's having an affair?'

I sipped my fake wine and hugged my knees into my chest. 'I don't know. I'm probably just being stupid, but,' I said

175

with a shrug, 'lately, it's just like we've been drifting apart. We never seem to have any time for each other anymore. I'm always caught in an anxious cycle – impatient until ovulation time, then pissed off when my period arrives. Part of me knows I'm pushing him away, but I've only been able to focus on one thing. It's worse than being addicted to drugs. Not that I ever have been, but, you know what I mean. It's like the worst kind of craving that never goes away. You eat, sleep, and breathe it constantly. It's an addiction. And the way I've been acting lately, I'm sure even you guys have been calling me Crazy Gina behind my back.'

Amelia chuckled. 'We've always called you Crazy Gina!'

'Yes, but that was crazy in a fun way. Now I'm crazy in a questionable-mental-health way.'

Kerry squeezed my arm gently. 'With all the treatment you've been through in the last few years, it's bound to put a lot of stress on both of you. Maybe you need to take some time out for yourselves after the IVF session. You know, spend more quality time together. I know it's easier said than done to forget about wanting a baby, but...' She gave me a sad smile, gauging my face for my reaction to what she was about to say. 'There has to be a cut-off point. A time when you say that's enough, and try to get on with your life.'

I nodded and glanced down at the floor. 'I know. I know you're right. Karl says the same thing, and I've started seeing this really lovely lady who does crystal healing, and she's given me lots to think about, too.' I told them all about Suzanne. 'You know Poppy's pregnant now, too.' I gave them a grim smile.

Stop it! Be genuinely happy! Wait for the good Karma to come back to you. Listen to Suzanne!

'Oh, honey.' Amelia put her arm round me and pulled me towards her so my head was resting against hers.

'But she was the one that gave me the idea about all this Universe stuff to begin with, and that's when I started talking to Zelda, and then I met Suzanne, and they gave me this idea...well, not *exactly* an idea, because I haven't got a clue what it means,' I said, aware that I was babbling.

Kerry and Amelia looked at me with confused expressions.

'I've been thinking a lot lately about how I'm going to need some new direction in my life. Just in case…you know, in case I can never get pregnant. I need something else to concentrate on to stop me falling apart. I have to break this vicious cycle I'm in.' I hesitated. 'Karl's been encouraging me to think about something, too.' I filled her in on Poppy and Suzanne's suggestion about asking the Universe for help, and being blown towards the travel agents, and how I thought it was a sign from Zelda.'

Surprisingly, they didn't even laugh. Maybe they were just being polite. If someone had said the same to me a year ago, I would've cracked up and dragged them off to the funny farm. Now I actually believed all this Universe stuff.

'Ooh, interesting,' Amelia released me and took a sip of her wine. 'But…how can that help you?'

'I don't know. Maybe that's what I'm supposed to do in life if I can't be a mum.' I shrugged.

'What? Go on holiday to Australia?' Kerry nodded thoughtfully, although she didn't look convinced. I wasn't convinced, either. I didn't know if this really was a sign, but I just had this weird feeling that Zelda meant me to see the travel agents. Or was I turning into a complete basket case? Maybe it was just an unexplainable mini tornado or something. Sometimes you got freak weather like that in the UK, didn't you?

'I agree you need some sort of project to get stuck into. Something new in your life to concentrate on to fill the gap,' Amelia said.

'I know.' I took another gulp of fake wine, contemplated stealing Amelia's real wine instead, and then set it back down on the floor. 'But a holiday's only a temporary fix. A two-week holiday isn't going to help me long term. It needs to be something drastic. A journey where I don't know what's going to happen.' I twisted round to face them. 'I think I want to travel around Australia for a while. Maybe a

177

year or so and see where we go from there. Take each day as it comes instead of being ruled by thermometers and periods. I need to get *me* back again, and Karl and I need to get back to appreciating each other before he really does get fed up with me and have an affair.'

'Wow!' Kerry rubbed her bump absentmindedly. 'That's definitely drastic!'

'What does Karl think?' Amelia exchanged a brief look of surprise with Kerry, as if worried I'd finally tipped over the edge.

'Erm…I haven't told him yet.'

'But what about his job – or your business, even?' Kerry asked.

'Yes, I'm not too sure about that part yet.' I waved my hand in the air. 'I haven't really thought about Karl's job. Obviously, I'd have to give up my clients, but maybe I could start something out there. I reckon with all that sunshine people will be *dying* for a Hollywood.' I giggled.

'God. I don't know what to say.' Amelia's eyes widened. 'I'll miss you if you go.'

'So will I! You're going to be a godmother soon,' Kerry said.

'Me, too.' I sniffed.

'But we're here to support you in anything you do. You know that, right?' Amelia gave me a concerned look.

I put my arms round both of them. 'Don't worry. I haven't gone completely off my trolley. And nothing is certain yet. I haven't even talked to Karl, so I don't know what will happen.'

Timetable City

My life was still being ruled by schedules. The day before, my period arrived, but I wasn't as angry as I'd been in the past. Now I had something else to concentrate on, I was feeling a whole lot more positive, plus, this time my period didn't mean the end of something. It meant the beginning of the IVF process.

As instructed, I had to phone the hospital to let them know, and they scheduled an appointment for me to pick up my fertility drugs. For the next few months my life would be:

Day 21 of cycle – Start down regulation drugs to suppress my natural hormones. I will have to sniff them twice a day, which will basically make my reproductive system shut down and send me spiralling into menopause.

2- 3 weeks later – 1st scan to check down regulation is working and look for any cysts. Apparently, cysts are a big side effect, and knowing my luck, I'll bloody well get them. *No, think positive. No cysts. None. Not even an ickle one.*

Start egg stimulation injections. Ew! An acupuncture needle wasn't as bad as expected, but the thought of sticking a needle in me is just horrible. A vision of all those butch nurses at school giving us our required jabs put me off for life.

7 - 8 days later – 2nd scan to check size of follicles/thickness of uterus.

5 - 10 days later – 3rd scan.

Final injection to start ovulation. Another one, yuck!

Thirty-five hours later – Egg collection. *Yes, it will work OK. I won't get stabbed in the bowel with the needle, or get an infection, or anything else for that matter.*

3 - 5 days later – Embryo transfer. *Ditto. And my embryos will be fully developed and fine because Zelda is going to make sure it happens. I trust you, Zelda. Pssst! Are you listening?*

I sorted out the drugs, some of which had to be stored in the fridge, and tried my hardest to forget about them, although that was easier said than done when I kept seeing them wedged in between the organic eggs and organic goat's milk every time I peered in for something to eat. The only way to take my mind off it was to get stuck into some research on Australia.

It had a population of around twenty-two million, and because most of it was desert or semi-desert, it had approximately two people per square kilometre of total land area. It was ranked seventeenth in the world for broadband uptake (always handy). It ranked 5th country in the world for beer drinking (Karl would be ecstatic). And it ranked thirty-third in the world for suicide rates. Oh, well, if my plans to travel around didn't work out we could always drink ourselves to death.

I perused the Australian Embassy's website and downloaded a couple of information packs. We were eligible to get a year's tourist visa to travel around. Perfect!

I scoured websites looking for pictures. Ayers Rock (I'd always been fascinated about that when I saw the film *Picnic at Hanging Rock* where the schoolgirls disappeared unexplainably. OK, so it was a completely different rock, but creepily fascinating, nevertheless), the Great Barrier Reef,

Sydney harbour, the outback (not too sure about that one, since I saw the film *A Cry in the Dark* where a dingo stole a baby), Tasmania (as long as I didn't bump into those little devils), the Gold Coast where we could pretend to be surfer dudes. The list of places to see and things to experience was amazing.

A bubble of excitement started at the pit of my stomach and worked its way up to my throat. Yes, this was it. We could hire out a campervan and just go where the whim took us, which was apparently a favoured way for travellers to sightsee. No more planning. No more stress. Just a chilled-out, healthy way of life, going from destination to destination, experiencing life again and being relaxed. If that didn't take my mind off things, I didn't know what would. And the possibilities were endless. We could fall in love with the place and decide to stay there. Some high-powered company might head-hunt Karl. I might win the National Brazilian Waxing Competition and be so in demand I'd have to turn clients away.

I stared out of the window and daydreamed. I could picture me in a bikini and Karl looking sexy in some tight trunks, instead of those horrible baggy boxers he'd been wearing. It was Christmas Day, and we were on the beach cooking turkey breasts on the barbie (had just learnt that's Australian for BBQ), instead of freezing to death round Dad and Lavinia's house because she was too tight to put the heating on. Karl and I both had golden tans, and I had a beautiful pink flower in my hair. Karl had a koala bear on his shoulder who was our pet (not entirely sure how we'd got him, but that wasn't important), and a couple of Aborigines were playing a didgeridoo around a camp fire.

I let out a blissful sigh.

We only had a small mortgage, so if we rented the house out, most of the money could go towards our travel expenses. We could live on a budget, act like teenagers again, and most importantly, have fun and appreciate what we had. Suzanne was always talking about living in the moment and taking the time to enjoy life. This was definitely the way to do it.

But what would Karl think about it?

Babies, Babies Everywhere

I still hadn't spoken to Karl about Australia. I wanted to make sure I knew as much as possible about it before I brought the possibility up so I could make it sound more appealing to him.

I'd started the nasal spray to down regulate my system and turn me into a cross between Mother Teresa and Arnold Schwarzenegger in *Terminator*. Even a simple trip to the supermarket was a nightmare. When a grungy teenager rammed his trolley into the back of my legs, I wanted to rip his head off and shove it down his throat. The next minute, I wanted to bring him home for tea and cook him a good meal. I'd avoided going out of the house ever since for fear of what might happen. It was like snorting cat's piss, and as well as the uncontrollable rages and mood swings, the other side effects were: headaches, night sweats, sneezeitis, knackerditis, and insomnia, which gave me plenty of time to surf the net on my quest to find out more about sunny Oz.

It was the weekend, and neither of us had work. Yippee! So I snuggled into Karl's shoulder as we lay in bed, wanting to stay there forever thinking nice, happy, positive thoughts, and daydreaming (which was my new favourite pastime) about which campervan we could hire out. Would we need a four-berth one, or would two be enough? They were pretty small, though. Would we feel claustrophobic? Should we fly to Sydney first or Perth?

I stared at his snoozing face and traced the contours of his nose gently with my finger. His dark brown hair was tinted with grey at the temples now, but he was still as gorgeous to me as when we first met.

We finally surfaced at 10 a.m., but he was in a really bored mood and kept pacing around aimlessly. I was trying to read *Marie Claire* but he kept putting me off, which was very annoying as there was an interesting article about a couple who travelled around the USA in a campervan for four years and had a blast.

I put my mug of peppermint tea down and watched him wandering around the lounge in a circle like a cat trying to catch its tail. 'What are you doing?'

'Thinking.' He clasped his hands together and pinched at his lips with his forefingers.

'What about?'

'Life.' He shrugged.

Well that narrowed it down a bit. 'Life in general, or something specific?' He was worrying me now. He had a funny kind of spaced out look on his face.

He stopped pacing and sank down next to me, opening his mouth to say something when the phone rang. 'I'll get it.' He leapt up and shot off into the hall.

I heard muffled conversation and strained my ears to eavesdrop but couldn't make much out.

'I'm going out.' He stuck his head round the door and sloped off again.

Was he acting weird, or was I imagining things?

One *Cosmo* and two *Marie Claires* later, Karl still wasn't back. Maybe he was organizing another surprise for my birthday. Or maybe he really was having a secret tryst with Britney. I was feeling restless myself, craving something, but not sure what. Chocolate? Wine? A cigarette? A shag? No, not a shag. I'd had enough to last a lifetime lately.

It couldn't be easy for him, either, could it? I knew he hated seeing me have to go through all the fertility treatment, and the worse bit was yet to come. I'd been too wrapped up in myself and how I was feeling to take notice of how difficult it must be for him to cope with not having a baby. Although he said he didn't mind whether we had a boy or a girl, I knew secretly he was longing to have a little boy to play with and do boys' stuff. The drugs were already messing up my system, and I was trying really hard not to take it out on him because he desperately felt the empty space of no children in our lives, too. I'd read a lot of stories about fertility treatment and IVF wrecking marriages. Did he want out of it? Would he leave me if I couldn't have a child?

Shut up brain! You mentioned the B-word. What did Suzanne tell you? Stop thinking about it and let it go.

Ha! That's easy for you to say!

It is easy because I'm your brain. Now pack it in!

Oh, fuck off, brain!

Ahem. That's no way to talk to me.

Maybe the cat's piss was giving me psychosis. Luckily, I was saved from any further schizophrenic tendencies by Mark phoning

'Kerry's had the baby!' He squealed down the phone. I didn't think it was possible for a man to squeal but there was definite squealing going on.

'And she'd love to see you all. If…' he paused for a minute. 'You know…if you want to.'

The thought of seeing and holding their baby filled me with dread for a moment, and I started having a mini panic attack. I'd have to hold it and pretend everything was OK; put on a brave face when all I wanted to do was hate Kerry and Mark. What if I couldn't control my jealousy? I wanted to kill someone. Kerry and Mark would do for starters. What if I was a complete bitch to them? What if I blubbed everywhere and embarrassed myself? What if it never happened for me? I had an overwhelming urge to throw up so I took some deep breaths before my brain started screaming at me again. Why did it all come so easy to Kerry who hadn't even wanted a baby? Why could she get pregnant on one stupid night when a condom split and I couldn't after months of timed-to-perfection sex?

That's when I heard Suzanne's voice in my head…

Success and happiness is infinite. Be genuinely happy for them. The happier you are, the more those things will come

185

to you. Trust that everything is connected. Visualize your baby and then let it go.

Then I felt so guilty. As usual, the hormones and obsession were taking over my rational thoughts. What was the point in feeling sorry for myself? It wasn't going to get me anywhere. And Suzanne was right. I needed to be positive. I had to get things into perspective. There were millions of starving people in the world. And what about the other millions dying from incurable diseases? At least I had enough food on the table, a shelter over my head, and I was healthy, even if my ovaries didn't seem to be functioning properly. It wasn't fair, but then who ever said life was fair? I didn't want Kerry to feel awkward or upset because she'd managed to do what I couldn't.

'When did she have it? Is it a girl or a boy? How much did it weigh?' I forced myself to sound happier.

'An hour ago. A girl. Seven and a half pounds. She's so beautiful.'

'Are they both OK?' I asked.

'Yes, they're both absolutely perfect. Can you ring Amelia and Dan and let them know? I want to get back to my family.' His voice was tinged with pride.

'Of course I will. And I'd love to come and see them,' I said. 'Now get off the phone and get back to them.'

Karl walked in as I was hanging up, thankfully not smelling of anything other than paint. He'd been helping Dan fit a new dongle-sprocket – or something or other – to his model train set.

'Kerry's had the baby,' I said, willing my voice to come out sounding happy. 'Let's go and visit her.' I grabbed my bag and rooted around for my car keys.

'Good for Kerry.'

I glanced up suddenly at the sadness in his voice. His shoulders sagged and his face had crumpled, making him look as worn out as I felt from all the lack of sleep.

'Oh, Karl.' I was overcome with a sinking feeling as I gathered him into my arms.

186

'I feel like I'm a failure,' he whispered into my hair. 'I can't give you what you want.'

'You're not a failure.'

He snorted.

'If anyone's a failure, it's me,' I said.

'When you first said you wanted a baby, I thought it would be easy. But the more time has gone on, and the more I see you go through all the treatment, it just makes me wonder what will happen if we can't have children. I know I'm not as emotionally involved in it all like you, but...' his voice cracked and I glanced up at him. Tears rolled freely from his bloodshot eyes. '...it doesn't mean I want it any less.'

'I know.' I stroked his back. 'Normally it's you that's the positive one, and I'm the negative one.'

'It seems like we've swapped places lately. I feel like I have to be the strong one all the time, but it's not easy for me, either.'

'Everything will work out OK. If it's meant to be, it will happen,' I said with more confidence than I actually felt, managing to raise a slight smile. If ever there was a time I needed to believe Suzanne, it was now. 'We'll get through this together.' I held onto him so tight I couldn't tell where his heartbeat began and mine ended.

As we walked along the hospital corridor towards Kerry's bed, I kept my eyes fixed on the floor in front of me so I wouldn't have to be confronted with the thing I wanted most in the world. Karl squeezed my hand beside me, acknowledging the sadness I felt inside. The sadness we both felt. I fully intended not to look at any of the ecstatic parents celebrating their good fortune, but the sound of a high-pitched wail jarred my head automatically in the direction of the cries. A woman was holding her baby, gazing down into its face with an expression of pure joy. A thought flitted through my brain for a brief moment – would anyone notice if I ran off with it? I glanced back down the corridor where we'd come from. No one was around. It would only take a couple of seconds to scoop up the baby and dash off. I could drive straight to Scotland. I'd dye my hair, wear a big bodysuit so I looked three stone heavier, dress in frumpy clothes. It was perfect. No one would recognize me…

'Gina?' Karl hissed, sending me tumbling back to reality as I realized I was rooted to the spot, still staring at the baby. I shook my head to clear it of irrational thoughts.

Kerry shifted into a sitting position in bed when we approached, a huge smile plastered on her face. 'Oh, I'm so glad you guys came.'

I bent over and hugged her. Karl slapped Mark on the back. To the outside world, we looked like we didn't have a care in the world.

I handed her a bunch of flowers we'd bought from the gift shop in the hospital. Even though there were baby clothes and accessories there, I couldn't bring myself to even pick them up, let alone buy them. 'Oh, she's so cute.' I smiled, but there was no joy in it.

Tucking my hair behind my ears, I leaned in over the clear plastic cot at the side of Kerry's bed. Nestled on a yellow blanket was the most beautiful baby I think I'd ever seen. She had huge blue eyes and a fine down of blonde hair.

'I know I'm biased.' Kerry laughed. 'But she's pretty drop-dead gorgeous.'

'Congratulations,' Karl said, hovering behind me, as if unsure what to do with himself.

Tears stung my eyes but I blinked them away. 'She's beautiful.'

Don't cry. Congratulate them and mean it. Be genuinely happy. It will project positive vibes back to you.

'So how are you feeling?' I asked Kerry, who looked exhausted but on a happy high.

She glanced down at her beautiful baby with a glowing smile that radiated pure love. 'I'm a bit sore, but she's worth it.'

A huge golf ball-sized lump formed in my throat but I forced it down as I reached out and put my little finger in the baby's tiny fist. With amazing strength, she squeezed back hard. Then she burped.

We all burst out laughing.

'I see she takes after her dad already,' Karl said.

'More like her mum, I'd say.' Mark grinned at Kerry and she tried to swipe him with her hand but he ducked out of the way.

'You can pick her up if you want.' Kerry glanced up at me nervously.

I looked at Karl for reassurance. I didn't know if it would make it worse, holding her in my arms.

You can do this.

I tentatively reached out, making sure I supported her head, and picked her up. She was warm and cuddly, and smelt of the unsullied pureness of new baby. As I held her to my chest, kissing her forehead gently, I felt like I was about to crack into a million pieces.

The Power of Life

The next few weeks passed by in such a rush I didn't have time to think much, which was definitely a good thing. I had clients coming out of my ears, booked solid because I was going to take it easy after the egg implant.

In between wanting to do a Mike Tyson impression and punch the shit out of people, or bawling my eyes out and wanting to hug everyone, I went to the hospital for various blood tests.

The night before my first scan, the phone rang off the hook with people wishing me luck.

First it was Dad. 'Hi, love. Just ringing to wish you lots of luck for tomorrow.'

'It's only a scan, don't worry. I'm sure everything will be fine,' I said with more confidence than I actually felt.

'Lavinia wanted me to wish you luck, too.'

Yeah, right. 'Tell her thanks.'

'Make sure you let me know how you get on, OK?'

'Will do. Love you.'

'Love you, too, sweetheart. Your mum would be proud of you, you know. You've turned into a wonderful woman,' he said, emotion filtering through his voice.

'Oh, Dad. Don't make me cry again! It doesn't take much these days.' I wiped my eyes, wishing Mum was still here to give me some moral support.

'Oh, sorry, pumpkin. OK, I'll get off the phone now.'

Then it was Poppy. 'I'm sending you positive vibes, Gina. And I've sent a message to the Universe to help you. I've got a good feeling about this.'

I smiled to myself. 'Thanks. Did your scans go OK? I

190

mean, I've had them before and I know they're not painful, but was everything going according to plan when you had your first scans after the down regulation drugs?' I couldn't stop worrying. What if I had a cyst? What if the drugs hadn't worked?

'Yes, everything was always going well at that stage. They'll probably tell you to start the injections next to stimulate your ovaries.'

'OK. Thanks for everything, Poppy. All the support you've given me, well...I don't know what I would've done without you.'

She chuckled. 'You're very welcome. Good luck.'

Then it was Amelia. 'Do you want me to come with you?'

'No, it's OK, but thanks for the offer. Karl's got to work, but it's not like he can do much at this stage, anyway.' I'd dealt with most of the other tests on my own. It wasn't like this was a biggie.

Unless they find a cyst or some other complication.

They won't. Shut up!

'Well ring me tomorrow and let me know what happens,' she said.

'I will.'

Then it was Kerry. 'I just wanted to say good luck. I'll be thinking of you.'

'Thanks. How's baby? Have you thought of a name yet?'

'We're going to call her Elise,' she said wistfully.

'I love it.'

'If you'd like to follow me,' a young nurse who looked about fifteen led me to the scanning room. She'd overdone it with the hot straighteners, and her hair was crispy like straw.

Was she old enough to be carrying out these tests? What if she was an imposter? Highly unlikely, I know, but my brain started going off on a worried tangent. What if she got the results wrong? What if she mixed up mine with someone else's? Obviously, she couldn't work a pair of simple hair straighteners, so how could she manage such complicated scanning equipment?

'OK, I just need you to pop your knickers off and get up on the couch.' She pulled a curtain to give me some privacy.

As I pulled off my knickers my rose quartz crystal that I'd completely forgotten about fell out and shot across the floor underneath the curtain.

'Shit,' I said, pulling my skirt down and peering out.

'What was that? Something just skidded across the floor.' The nurse was bending down under the scanning equipment, trying to get a look at the offending article.

'Er…it's a crystal.' I cringed, flushing with embarrassment at how ridiculous I must seem to her.

She glanced up at me sympathetically. 'Don't worry. I've seen all sorts of lucky charms in here.' She wheeled the machine out of the way and I grabbed the crystal and put it in my bag for safekeeping.

I lay back on the couch as she performed the scans, pointing at something on the screen occasionally to show another nurse who'd joined us. I craned my neck, trying to get a look but it all looked like a big, blobby mess to me.

'Does everything look OK?' I asked about a million times.

'Everything looks fine,' the fifteen-year-old said.

'What's that?' I pointed to a dark patch on the screen. 'That doesn't look OK.'

'That's your kidney,' she said.

'Right. So everything's OK?'

She returned the transducer to its socket and gave me some tissues to clean off the gel. I could've sworn I heard her sigh, though.

What? Just checking. You're only fifteen, what do you know?

'Everything is absolutely fine,' she repeated slowly, as if talking to a five-year-old. 'Now we need you to start taking the follicle stimulating hormone injections.' She handed me a slip of paper with instructions on. 'You'll do one every day, injected in the fleshy part of your stomach. Pop your knickers on and stand up and I'll show you what you need to do.' She pulled the curtain back around me and I obliged.

'Just pull the top of your skirt down,' she said. 'OK, here.' She grabbed a wobbly bit of flesh just underneath my belly button and pressed it together. 'This is where you need to inject.' Then she got the injection pen and showed me how to work it. 'The pens are pre-filled with three doses in them, so one pen will last three days.'

I pulled a face. 'Does it hurt?'

She smiled. 'No.'

Hmmm. I wasn't convinced about that.

She started writing something down in her notes. 'I've booked you another scan in five days time so we can check how you're getting on.'

'Right, thanks. And you're sure everything's OK?'

'Yes!'

I was staring at the injector pen when Karl came home. It looked pretty much like a regular pen. Harmless, innocuous. But it was what was inside it that counted. This drug had the power to create life.

'Hey, that's good news about the scan, isn't it? Everything's going OK.' He kissed me on the cheek. 'Have you done it yet?' He nodded towards the pen.

'No. I'm scared.'

He rubbed my shoulders. 'Do you want me to do it for you?'

'Would you?'

'Well, I wouldn't exactly enjoy it. It would freak me out, actually, sticking a needle in you, but if you want me to, I'll give it a go.'

I carried on staring at it. *Oh, for God's sake, don't be such a wimp!* 'Yeah, I know what you mean. I don't think I could stick one in you, either. Although, to be honest, I have felt like it on many occasions lately.' I chuckled as I clutched it in my hand. 'Probably the thought of doing it is worse than actually doing it. What do you think?' I glanced at him for encouragement.

'Absolutely. I bet you won't even feel a thing.' He nodded vigorously.

I pulled the protective cap off the top and stared at the needle. I was expecting some huge thing, but it was actually quite small. I pulled the top of my skirt down, squashed a couple of inches of flesh between my fingers and hovered the needle over it.

'Right. Here goes,' I said.

'I can't look.' He slapped a hand over his eyes.

'That's not making me feel any better,' I said. 'Maybe I shouldn't look either.' I squeezed my eyes shut.

'Yeah, but what if you stick it somewhere else by accident?' he said.

Damn. Good point.

I opened my eyes, took a deep breath, and slid the needle into my skin. Only a slight prick. So far so good. I clicked the top of the pen to release the dose and slid the needle back out slowly.

'Have you done it yet?' Karl asked.

'Yep,' I said, feeling pretty proud of myself. 'The fear of doing it is the biggest hurdle. It really didn't hurt at all.'

He dropped his hand away from his eyes. 'Well done,' Karl repeated over and over. 'I can't believe you did it.'

Two days later, I'd just done my third injection and pulled the needle out when I noticed there was still a decent amount of the liquid left in the syringe. That didn't make sense, though, because the nurse told me I had enough for three days so why was there some left over?

I pulled back on the top of the pen to check how much was actually in there and accidentally squirted out what was left inside onto the kitchen table.

Oh, shit! What am I supposed to do now?

The pen should've been empty, but it wasn't, which sent me into full-scale panic mode. I couldn't have been giving myself the right dose. What if the drugs didn't work because of it? Should I give myself another injection now? What if

I'd screwed up the whole treatment? Would I have to start all over again?

I quickly phoned the hospital and breathlessly explained what had happened.

'It's OK, Gina,' Scottish Claire said to me. 'The pens are prefilled with a little extra dosage, that's all. It's natural to have some left in them when you've finished the three days.'

'So it will still work OK, then? I have been doing it right?'

'Yes. Don't panic, Gina. Everything's fine.'

My shoulders relaxed with relief.

Hope

Two days later, I was back for my next scan. I was so nervous I started hyperventilating on the train on the way to the hospital, and my palms were sweaty.

The fifteen-year-old nurse had been replaced by Claire, which made me feel slightly more at ease. She led me into the small treatment room as I tried to calm myself down.

Zelda, it's me again. Can you please, please, please make sure everything's going according to plan?

'We're doing a transvaginal scan today, so off with your knickers and get yourself comfy on the couch.' She gave me a warm smile. 'I'll be back with the doctor.'

I lay back, staring at the ceiling, twiddling with the blanket covering me for what seemed like an eternity until a tiny Indian doctor came in.

'Hello, Gina. How are you today?' she asked.

Stressed! Hurry up and tell me what's going on. 'Fine, thanks.'

'Any side effects from the injections?'

Yes, I'm going to punch you if you don't hurry up! 'Well, the mood swings are pretty bad.'

She patted my arm and smiled. 'That's normal.' She pulled on some rubber gloves. 'Now, let's have a look. Put your feet together and drop your knees to the side for me, please.' She slid a condom on the giant willy probe and inserted the fufu cam, then turned back to the screen on the scanner.

I tried to look, then turned my head away and concentrated on the rest of the equipment in the room to take my mind off feeling anxious.

One set of scales.

Three models of fufus.

A sharps bin.

Something that looked like toilet roll for an elephant, although I suspected it was to cover the couch with.

Then I couldn't help myself anymore and turned to look at the screen. I could see some round things on there but I didn't know if that was good or bad.

The doctor clicked the scanner machine and it took stills of the screen. Then she put markers on different points of the blobs and the machine calculated the size of them.

'What do you think, Doctor?' I asked, about to burst with anticipation.

'It's all looking very good. You've got eight follicles forming.' She smiled and removed the fufu cam. 'I'll need to do another scan in five days.'

Thank God I had a crystal healing session booked the next day. I needed a severe dose of relaxation, and I needed Suzanne to keep me sane.

'The mood swings are bad enough, but I just feel so restless,' I told Suzanne. 'And I know you're going to say I'm not living in the moment, but I can't right now. I've been really good, taking on board everything you said, but I'm just worried all the time and I can't seem to relax.'

The corners of her eyes crinkled as she smiled. 'Of course you feel like that. It's all the drugs and the stress. Not everyone can cope with IVF so I think you should be incredibly proud of yourself.'

I relaxed as she said that. How was it she always knew exactly what to say to make me feel better?

'Part of me feels hope, too,' I said. 'Hope that it's going to work out, but part of me feels overwhelming fear that it won't.'

'Have you thought about meditating?'

'I tried some relaxation CDs before but they didn't do anything except stress me out.' I let out an ironic laugh.

'Gina, Gina, Gina, what am I going to do with you?' She

197

shook her head good-naturedly. 'Mahatma Ghandi said, "What you think, you become," which is pretty true. Meditation lets you clear your thoughts completely so your brain has time to rest. We have all these thoughts bombarding us all the time so we need to take time out. Think of your brain as a computer. If you don't clear out the clutter every now and then, the hard disk gets full up and doesn't work properly. Taking five or ten minutes a day with no thoughts in your head can make all the difference to your stress levels and ability to cope with life.'

'My husband would think I was really crazy if I sat on the lounge floor chanting *Om* all the time.' I rolled my eyes at her.

She laughed. 'All our fears and worries are just thoughts.' She shrugged. 'Purely and simply, that's what they are. Meditation can help let them go. Get them to disappear completely. You don't have to chant anything if you don't want to. Simply concentrating on your breathing, or listening to music, or cleaning can be meditation. As long as you clear your mind of the clutter and distraction by not thinking, it can be effective.'

'I know me, though. As soon as I try not to think about something, I think about it more.'

'I know. It takes practice. At first, when you try to clear your mind, you'll find all these thoughts rushing in, but after you've done it a few times you'll learn how to push them away.'

'OK, tell me what I need to do,' I said.

After dinner that night I sneaked up to the bedroom so Karl wouldn't ask me what I was doing. I dimmed the lights, sat on the floor with my legs crossed and my back against the wall and closed my eyes.

I concentrated on my breathing. In. Out. In. Out.

My brain carried on thinking in overdrive.

Will it work?

Will we travel to Australia?

Will Karl and I stay together?

Can I cope with not being a mother?

My fears and worries are just thoughts. My fears and worries are just thoughts.

And then, I repeated a word over and over again in time to my breathing.

Hope. Hope. Hope.

I heard Karl's footsteps at the top of the hallway. As he made his way into the bedroom I expected him to crack up with laughter, but I didn't open my eyes.

'What are you doing?' he asked.

'Meditating.'

Hope. Hope. Hope.

He sat down on the floor next to me and I opened one eye to see what he was up to. He had his legs crossed, too.

'So what do you have to do?' he asked.

'Try and concentrate on nothing. Repeat a word over again in time to your breathing to clear your mind.'

'What word are you using?'

'Hope,' I said softly, peering at him with one open eye.

'OK.' He reached out and cupped my cheek in his hand. 'I love you.'

I smiled. 'I love you, too.'

He closed his eyes, a grin forming in the corner of his lips. 'If you tell anyone I'm doing this, I'll kill you.'

Operation Ejaculation

I don't know if it was the meditation or not, but I was feeling a bit calmer by the time I went for my next scan. Unless you count a little episode where I kicked the stainless steel bathroom bin because Karl squeezed the toothpaste from the middle of the tube instead of the end. Now I had what looked more like a steel drum than a practical bathroom item.

'Excellent,' the little Indian doctor said as she examined my follicles again on the scanner. 'They're just the right size.'

'Wow!' Relief flooded my veins. 'That's fantastic.'

She glanced at the clock. It was 1.00 p.m. 'At one o' clock in the morning you need to do the injection of HCG, which completes the final maturation of the follicles and loosens the egg's attachment from the follicle wall.' She scribbled down some notes. 'We need to do the egg collection thirty-five hours after the injection. So we need you here for half-past eleven on Thursday morning.'

I glanced at her wide-eyed with excitement. This was it. After all this time, it's what I'd been waiting for. 'Oh, my God. I can't believe it.' I threw my arms around her and hugged her tight.

She patted my back and extricated herself slowly, smiling. 'Your husband can either do his sperm donation here at the hospital, or if you live within two hours away, he can do it at home and you can bring it with you.'

I didn't think Karl would be too impressed about doing it at the hospital again after the last time. 'I'll need a pot, please.'

'Here you go.' She handed me one in a sealed bag.

'Double wow!' I said, taking it off her, still in shock. 'I have to ring my husband.' I rushed to get dressed and get out of there so I could tell him the fantastic news.

'Wowwwwwwwwwwwwwww!' I screamed down the phone at him.

'That's great. Not long to go now.' I heard the smile in his voice.

'I can't believe it. We're finally getting the chance to be parents.' I giggled, ignoring the strange looks I was getting from patients coming into the hospital. 'And I got you a pot to use.'

'Oh, damn. And I so wanted to do it in a broom cupboard again.'

When I got home, I scoured the train timetable online. This had to be the most precision timed wank of all. If Karl did the sperm sample too early, it might be ruined by the time we got to the hospital, and if we arrived at the hospital too late, I might've already ovulated, and once that happened, my eggs couldn't be retrieved and we would miss our chance. Talk about pressure for Karl! I jotted down everything and double-checked it about twenty times:

Need a lift from the house to station – 09.45 a.m.
Train leaves station – 10.01 a.m.
Train arrives King's Cross – 10.31 a.m.
Allow a ten minute walk to tube station – 10.46 a.m.
Allow a ten minute wait for tube – 10.56 a.m.
Ten minutes on tube – 11.06 a.m.
Twelve minutes to walk to hospital – 11.16 a.m.
Two minutes in lift – 11.18 a.m.

Right. So that meant Operation Ejaculation had to be carried out by 9.44 a.m.

I reached for the phone and called Dad.

'Hey, pumpkin. How are you?'

'I've got eight follicles!' I gushed.

'Wow, that's fantastic. I'm so happy for you. When are they doing the egg retrieval?'

'In three days, which is why I'm calling. We need a lift to the station, but it has to be timed exactly because of Karl's sperm.'

'OK. Let me just grab a pen, hang on a sec.' I heard him rustling papers before he came back on the phone. 'Right. What time do you need me to pick you up?'

'Nine forty-five exactly. If you're early, can you just wait on the drive and we'll come out. I don't want Karl to have any interruptions at the crucial moment.'

'Right you are. Don't worry, love. Everything's going to be fine.'

'Karl,' I whispered in the darkness at midnight.

'What?' He turned over.

'I've just checked the injection I have to do and there's a humongous needle on the end of it. Do you think I'm supposed to stick it all the way in? It's massive!'

He rolled over and turned on the lamp, rubbing his eyes.

'Look, it's about two inches!'

'Bloody hell!' His eyes focused on it.

'I know. They didn't mention anything about that.' I glanced nervously at the clock. 'There won't be anyone there now to ask. Shall I pop down to Accident and Emergency and ask someone if it's OK? I don't want to pierce my stomach or something by doing it.'

He flipped the covers back. 'Come on. I'll drive you.'

I paced the floor of the accident and emergency department while the nurse paged an on call gynaecologist to come down and speak to us. I looked at my watch every couple of minutes. What if I went past the 1 a.m. scheduled time to inject the HCG? Would it be OK, or would the whole treatment be ruined? Would months of planning and waiting be wasted? I gnawed on my thumbnail.

Finally, she managed to get hold of someone.

'The injection needs to be done into your muscle,' the

gynaecologist said. 'That's why there's a longer needle on it. Just do it in your stomach where you've been doing the others, but be aware it might be sore for a few days.'

I groaned inwardly for a second. My stomach was already a patchwork of bruises from the injections.

'Thanks so much for your help!' I cried, already half way out the door so we could get back home and administer it.

Two Eggs and Chips

I couldn't sleep the night before the egg retrieval. I tried to meditate. I tried to concentrate on my breathing and relax. I even tried warm goat's milk but nothing was working. I felt sick with worry about the procedure, which Poppy had said was pretty painful. Would something go wrong? Would they get the eggs OK? Would they fertilize?

But at the same time I felt hope. This was my final chance to get pregnant. So far, everything had gone well. Who was to say the rest of it wouldn't, as well? In a couple of weeks, I could be holding my baby in my arms like Kerry.

Zelda! Are you there? It will work, won't it?

Zelda?

Why can't you just answer me instead of sending signs?

I turned over in bed for the gazillionth time, huffing.

'Karl, are you awake?' I poked his shoulder at four o'clock in the morning.

No response.

How could he sleep at a time like this? Didn't he realize how scary and exciting this was?

'Karl.' I poked him harder. 'Are you awake?'

'I wasn't, but it looks like I am now.'

'Will it work?' I asked.

'Uh-huh.'

'What does that mean? Is that a yes or no?'

'Yes,' he insisted.

'Why don't we get up now in case we oversleep and miss the alarm? The batteries might run out overnight and we might miss the train,' I said, picking up the clock next to my bed to check it was still working.

'I've set the alarm on my phone, too. Go back to sleep. You need to get some rest.'

I plumped up my pillow, lifted myself up onto my elbow and rested my head in my hand. 'I can't sleep.'

'Well, I can.' He turned his back on me.

Bloody cheek!

'How do men do that? How can men sleep when there's something stressful going on?' I sighed.

'It's one of our amazing attributes. Like women can multi-task. We can sleep.'

'Well, it's not fair.' I poked him again. 'So, anyway. What time do you think you'll have to start masturbating to ejaculate at 9.44 a.m.? Do you want me to help?'

'Gina!' he grabbed his pillow and pulled it over his head. 'I'm not going to start bashing one out now so leave me alone. You'll be entering me into the wanking Olympics next!'

'What if there's a train strike?' I ignored him and carried on.

'There won't be,' his muffled voice groaned.

'But how do you know?' I said, aware that I was being annoying but the timing was absolutely crucial. I hadn't come all this way and gone through all this horrible treatment, not to mention emotional trauma, to have it ruined by something out of my control. 'What about a derailment? That could mess everything up.'

'Stop thinking about it.'

'What if there's an inconsiderate suicide bomber on the tube?'

'Suicide bombers are only human. Once we explained our predicament, I'm sure they'd understand and let us be on our way.' He threw the pillow at me. 'Turn over.'

'Why?'

'Well, the only way *I'm* going to get any sleep is if *you're* asleep. So turn over and I'll give you a back massage.'

'Ooh, I like the sound of that.' I turned over as his hands went to work, kneading my shoulders.

'What's this?' Karl noticed the drawstring bag from the spell I'd done, poking out from under my pillow. He pulled it out, frowning at it.

'Nothing.' I gave him a sheepish look.

He undid it and peered inside. 'A pink stone and a bit of smelly stick.' He held it up, eyebrow raised. 'Do we have to sleep on a bed filled with garden rubbish now? What have you put under my pillow? A dog's turd from the local park?'

I snatched it off him, embarrassed. 'It's that spell I did, OK?'

He tried to suppress a snort but it didn't work. 'A spell? I thought you were joking when you told that couple at the hospital open evening. Haven't we got enough with one witch in the family?'

'It's a real fertility spell, actually.'

'And you seriously think this ridiculous idea will work?' He gave me a disbelieving look.

'There was a woman on Fertility Friends who did one and got pregnant straight away.' I heard my voice becoming defensive.

He shook his head. 'If someone had suggested you did a spell before all this baby business started you would've thought they were nuts.'

'I know, but I need all the help I can get.'

'I'm not saying anything,' he said in a tone of voice that said it all.

We finally got up at half past seven and had breakfast. Well, Karl had breakfast. I just played with my organic wholemeal toast and organic strawberry jam. Every time I went to take a bite, I felt nauseous.

'You should finish your breakfast. You won't be able to eat anything after this because of the sedative.' Karl tucked into a couple of boiled eggs.

I averted my eyes, the thought of eggs bringing about a fresh wave of anxiety. 'I'm not hungry.'

I glanced at the clock again. Only a minute had gone past

since the last time. I stood up and paced the floor.

At half-past nine, I had my coat on and Karl was reading a report from work.

'Are you going to start?' I asked him.

'Hmm?' he glanced up at me.

I mimed a wanking action. 'It's half nine. You know what happened last time at the hospital. It took you ages.'

'That's because I was in a broom cupboard!'

'Do you want a hand?' My eyes darted nervously to his crotch. 'You've only got fourteen minutes to do it before we have to leave.'

'No. I think at the moment you'd put me off with all your nerves flying around.'

'So go on then!'

'Yes, sir, Sergeant Major, sir!' He leapt up and saluted me, then grabbed the pot from the kitchen side.

I tapped my watch and he rolled his eyes at me and disappeared upstairs.

I looked at the clock. 9.33 a.m. He had twelve minutes left. I thought I was going to throw up.

I grabbed a glass of water and downed it.

9.34.

I stared out of the window and saw Dad pull up on the drive, hoping Karl hadn't heard it in case it put him off.

I sat down, resting my head in my hands and jigging my legs up and down. Then I stood up and paced the floor.

9.38.

He should've started earlier. I knew it! Why was I the only one panicking around here?

At 9.43 he came downstairs with a big smile on his face and handed me the pot. 'There.'

I shoved it down the top of my leggings. 'Dad's here. We might as well go.' I grabbed Karl's jacket and thrust it towards him.

Dad knocked at the door.

'Hang on a sec, I just need to get something.' Karl went into the lounge and came back with a big silver milk churn we used as an ornament.

'What are you doing?' I hissed.

He grabbed a label from the office desk, wrote *Karl's Sperm Sample* on it and stuck it on the front of the huge churn. Then he opened the door and held it up to Dad who stood on the doorstep. 'Can you give me a hand with this?'

Dad rushed to take it off him. 'Ah, right. That's your…erm…'

Karl burst out laughing.

I rolled my eyes at Karl, grinning in spite of how stressed I felt. 'Come on!' I put the churn back in the house and slammed the door. 'Stop mucking about.'

Dad chuckled. 'You've got plenty of time, love. Don't panic.'

On the train en route to London we didn't speak. I couldn't. I was too busy freaking out inside. I was very conscious of Karl's sperm down the front of my leggings. How weird it was to think that I was on my way to getting pregnant but the sperm was on the outside of my uterus, instead of the inside. This wasn't exactly how I'd envisioned getting pregnant all those months ago. A candle-lit dinner with a nice bottle of wine, or a cosy little holiday for two, followed by romantic love-making, yes. In a hospital, with a test tube, definitely a no-no. It felt so clinical and disconnected – the most unromantic thing in the world.

I tried to shield the pot carefully in case someone accidentally bumped into me and broke the container. One little slip and everything could go wrong.

I stared out of the window at the world speeding by. In a distant field, I spotted two magpies. They were supposed to be lucky, weren't they? What was the saying? One for sorrow, two for joy? That had to be a good sign.

I reached for Karl's hand and he gripped it like he never wanted to let me go.

****

208

'You can put your bag and clothes in here.' Claire showed us to a cubicle with a bed and locker next to it. 'Then put your gown on.' She nodded to a blue gown on the bed with ties at the back. 'Have you got the sperm specimen?'

'Yes.' I pulled it out of my leggings and handed it over.

She wrote Karl's name, date of birth, and the time it was taken on it, then hurried off.

I got undressed and Karl did up the ties on my gown with fumbling hands.

Half an hour later, the embryologist arrived. She was tall and slim and glamorous, and looked more like a catwalk model than someone who'd be popping eggs out of me.

'Hi, I'm Dr Sheena Coulson. I'll be doing the egg retrieval for you today.' She smiled at us and examined some notes on her clipboard. 'Do you want to go in with Gina?' she asked Karl.

He looked at me to see what I wanted.

I nodded at him.

'Yes.'

'OK, we'll take you down in about fifteen minutes and get everything set up.' She shook our hands and disappeared.

More intolerable waiting until the anaesthesiologist arrived. 'I'm Dr Jones, and I'll be administering the sedative for you today.' More note examining. 'Do you have any allergies to any medication?'

'Not that I know of,' I said.

'OK. We just need a signature on this consent form.' He handed me a form on a clipboard and I squiggled my signature on it. 'See you soon.' And he was gone.

When Claire came to get me, I'd had about ten nervous wees. She wheeled me on a stretcher into a room with lots of futuristic medical instruments and machinery that looked like something out of a scary science fiction film.

I gulped, my eyes darting from the equipment to Karl and back again.

He bit his lip, holding onto my hand.

Opposite me, there was what looked like a small dinner

hatch in the side of the wall that you'd find in a café.

The hatch suddenly flew open and a plump nurse with grey hair peered her head through.

The whole thing seemed so surreal I just blurted out, 'Two egg and chips please.'

Karl laughed next to me.

I grew hot with embarrassment and slapped a hand over my mouth when I realized I'd said it out loud, worrying that a sudden onset of Tourette's was another side effect of the hormones.

Everyone else chuckled, as if trying to humour a nervous, hormonal woman.

'Can I have your name and date of birth, please,' the dinner lady said through the hatch.

I gave her my details.

She nodded and handed something to Dr Coulson.

When everyone had stopped checking their equipment, Dr Jones gave me a sedative, and I passed out. Well, I sort of passed out. I could hear myself groaning in pain. God, Dr Dye had nothing on this lot. It was bloody agony, like someone was repeatedly stabbing my insides with knives.

I came round properly back in the cubicle in a lot of pain. 'Ouch.' I opened my eyes and Karl leaned forward, resting his elbows on the bed, his face the colour of raw cake mixture.

'Are you OK?' he asked.

'No. I could feel it when they were doing it. It still hurts.' I slurred, rubbing my stomach.

'This is crazy. You shouldn't have to be going through this. It was horrible to see you in so much pain.' His voice overflowed with anger and passion.

I squeezed his hand again. 'How many eggs did they get?'

'Five.' He rubbed my arm and kissed my cheek.

'Only five? They said I had eight follicles.'

Just then, I heard the woman in the next cubicle tell her husband they got seventeen eggs and I felt like the IVF idiot. If I wasn't still half doped up and in agony, I would have marched around the curtain and punched her lights out.

'God, I feel sick,' my mouth started watering and my stomach churned. 'Can you tell the nurse?'

Karl rushed off and came back with a nurse who had a cardboard kidney-shaped sick bowl in her hand.

'Don't feel well.' I struggled onto my side and threw up in the bowl.

'You may be having a reaction to the pethidine,' the nurse said. 'I'll give you an anti-sickness injection.' She disappeared off again as I puked for England.

When she returned she gave me an injection in my bum. 'That should get you feeling a bit better.'

'You look green.' Karl's eyes moistened with tears.

'I feel green,' I croaked before throwing up again. 'Can I have some water?' I wiped my mouth with tissues and he poured some water from a jug on the locker.

I lay on my side, Karl stroking my back as finally the sickness subsided.

When the nurse came back, she suggested Karl go and get me something to eat to help settle my stomach.

'What shall I get you?' Karl asked me.

'Ugh! I don't want to eat anything,' I said.

'How about a sandwich?' the nurse suggested.

'OK.' It was easier to agree than resist.

Half a sandwich, a pint of water, and an hour later I was feeling a bit more human, although still in pain, drained, and tired. 'I want to go home,' I told Karl, although I was dreading the train journey on the way back.

On wobbly legs, I got dressed as Karl supported me.

Claire returned and cut off my hospital wristband. 'Take it easy on the way home. If you have any problems, give us a ring. We'll phone you tomorrow to give you an update on the fertilization.' She gave me a sympathetic smile. 'Good luck, Gina. I've got my fingers crossed for you.'

Karl put me to bed when I got home and I was off in la la land as soon as my head hit the pillow. It was the first decent sleep I'd had in ages, although that was probably due to the drugs still in my system. I didn't even hear Karl get up the next morning and woke up at 10 a.m. when he brought me a cup of green tea.

'Have they phoned yet?' I asked him when he sat on the edge of the bed.

He pursed his lips and shook his head.

'I wonder when they'll ring,' I said.

'Hopefully soon. How're you feeling?'

'Like someone's been shoving knitting needles up my fufu.'

'Do you want some pain killers? They said you can have some.'

'No, thanks,' I said as the phone next to Karl's side of the bed rang.

I looked at him.

He looked at me.

Then he dived for the phone.

'Hello?' He answered the phone as my heartbeat clanged around in my chest. There was a pause, then: 'Oh, hi.' He glanced at me and mouthed, "It's your dad." 'She's a bit sore, but OK. Do you want to talk to her?' He passed the phone to me.

'Are you OK, pumpkin?' Dad asked.

'Yes, I'm fine. Just a bit sore. Listen, sorry Dad, but the hospital might be trying to get through to tell me if the eggs have fertilized.'

'Oh, OK. Ring me later, then, when you find out. I've got my fingers crossed.'

I hung up and it immediately rang again. I stared at the phone in my hand and passed it to Karl. 'You answer it. I'm scared.'

He answered, then rolled his eyes at me. 'Hi, Amelia. No, she's fine, but we're waiting for a phone call from the hospital. Uh-huh. Yes. I'll get her to ring you later.' He hung up.

Three agonizing hours later, they phoned. I heard Karl's

212

voice downstairs as he answered. Then his heavy footsteps as he ran up the stairs.

He burst in the bedroom door, a massive smile on his face. 'Two eggs have fertilized.'

My hands shot to my mouth and I burst into tears. 'Oh, my God!'

Come to Mama

Two days later, we were back at the hospital for the embryo transfer.

I stopped short in front of the entrance doors. 'I can't believe this is happening.' I felt a surreal glow inside. My eggs fertilized. They actually fertilized, and I'd had a permanent smile on my face since I got the news.

'We're going to be parents.' Karl picked me up and spun me around, oblivious to all the other people coming and going. 'This is going to work. I've got a great feeling about it.'

'Agh! Put me down. You're making me dizzy.' I giggled.

'Sorry.' He released his hold on me.

I stood staring up at the hospital where our embryos were being stored. Our babies. There are events in your life that are so profoundly important they can be categorized as either pre-event or post-event. This was one of them. Before I stepped through that door, I wasn't pregnant. When I stepped out, I'd have my two little beans inside me, waiting to start their life. I was scared and happy and excited all at once.

'Are you ready to go in?' Karl took my hand, smiling down at me.

Come on babies. Come to mama.

I nodded. 'Yep. I've been ready for nearly two years.'

I was back in a cubicle again in one of the sexy hospital gowns. Everyone said the embryo transfer wasn't a painful procedure, but then they'd said I'd only feel some cramps with the HCG and egg retrieval and they were agony, so I was still nervous about what to expect.

214

'The doctor will be in to talk to you about your embryos in a minute,' Claire said as I looked at my watch for the hundredth time.

'Thanks.' I smiled and took some deep breaths.

'I'm really proud of you, Gina.' Karl reached for my hand. 'You're so strong and determined. You go for everything you want with such energy. You're going to be a fantastic mum.'

'Oh, stop it. You'll make me cry, and I don't want to cry today.' I hugged him, feeling tears prick behind my eyelids.

Luckily, he was saved from making me more emotional by the arrival of the doctor.

'Hi, I'm Dr Swanson, your reproductive endocrinologist.' A middle-aged woman with straight black hair poked her head around the cubicle curtain.

I repeated her name in my head because I wanted to remember the name of the woman who implanted my embryos forever. I'd have her to thank when it all worked out.

'What's your first name?' I asked her, thinking I could name the baby after her out of gratitude.

'Maude,' she said, sitting down on the corner of my bed.

OK, maybe not, then.

'How are you feeling?' she asked me.

'Nervous and excited.' I grinned.

She grinned back and nodded. 'Let me tell you a little bit about your embryos.' She glanced down at a folder of notes she had in her hand and pulled out a small picture of two round blobs that looked a bit like flowers. 'This is a picture of them.' She handed it to me and Karl stood over my shoulder to get a better look. 'By now we would've liked to see them divide into at least eight cells, but yours haven't.'

I took a sharp breath, hearing the suck of air through my mouth. 'Oh, so that's bad, then?' My voice came out high with astonishment.

'One of your eggs is still at the four-cell stage and one is at six cells, which means they're a little underdeveloped. The

215

important thing to remember is that women give birth to healthy babies all the time when they're implanted with a six-cell embryo, so there's still a fantastic chance of a successful pregnancy. Four-cell embryos have also gone on to produce a live birth, but realistically they have a lower chance of implantation,' she said.

'Oh.' My jaw dropped and I blinked at her. I didn't know what to say. I looked at Karl, who looked as devastated by the news as I felt.

'I just want to be clear,' Karl said firmly. 'You're not saying it won't work if you transfer them? It could still work, even though they're underdeveloped?'

She smiled. 'Yes, it could still work. As I said, it's perfectly possible you'll achieve a live birth with them.' She looked at me. 'I'd recommend we perform the embryo transfer as planned.'

I stared at the picture I held in my hand, feeling an overwhelming attachment to them. They were ours. Karl's and mine. I certainly hadn't come all this way to turn down my embryos just because they were a little bit underdeveloped. We still had a fighting chance, and boy was I going to take it.

'Yes, I want to go ahead.' I nodded enthusiastically.

'Good.' She stood up. 'I'll see you in a few minutes, then.'

When she left, Karl sat on the bed and hugged me. 'It will work. I know it will. So what if they're underdeveloped? As long as they've got your fighting spirit, they'll be fine.' He stroked my shoulder.

'Of course it will work.' I tried to push out all the worries and negative thoughts that seemed to be suddenly invading my brain.

Fears and worries are just thoughts. I don't want you in my head so bugger off! It will work.

A few minutes later, I was back in the same room with the serving hatch, lying on my back with Karl clutching my hand for dear life as we looked at Dr Swanson and the nurse arranging more space age equipment and something that

216

looked like a turkey baster.

'Ouch,' I said to him as his grip got harder.

He loosened it. 'Oh, God, sorry.'

'Are you ready?' Dr Swanson turned to me.

I nodded vigorously.

'I'm going to insert a speculum first of all, then we'll use a solution to clear any cervical mucus that may hinder the placement of the embryos.'

I grinned up at Karl with excitement.

Claire put some gel on my stomach and rubbed an ultrasound scanner head over it. 'This is so Dr Swanson can accurately implant the embryos into the best position,' she said.

I craned my neck, looking at the scanning machine to get a bird's-eye view of seeing them when they went in.

'I'm just inserting the catheter that contains the embryos into your cervix and up into your uterus.' Dr Swanson carried on looking at the screen, and I saw the catheter/turkey baster going in. 'Just going to find the best position for them.'

I stared at the screen, fascinated until she said, 'I'm going to release them from the catheter now.'

Karl resumed his vice-like grip on my hand. I squeezed back.

'And there they are.' She pointed at the fuzzy black and white screen, but I couldn't see much.

'We'll give you an ultrasound picture to take with you.' Claire smiled at us.

'Oh, wow, thanks,' I said. The second picture of our babies in one day. How amazing was this!

'OK, you need to keep lying down and rest for two hours before you can go home,' Dr Swanson said. 'You should take it easy for the first couple of days. That means no heavy lifting, no strenuous activity. No hot baths or swimming pools. No intercourse and no orgasms until we know the results of the pregnancy test.'

'So I don't need to rest in bed for the first two days?' I

asked.

'No, but definitely take it easy,' she said. 'After the first couple of days you can return to work, as long as it doesn't require lifting, being immersed in water, or physical exertion. You can also do light housework and drive.'

'Gotcha,' I said, thinking I might spend the first two days in bed, anyway, just to be on the safe side.

'And you'll need to insert the vaginal progesterone suppositories every night from tonight onwards. You may get some spotting or cramps. Spotting can be from the catheter, which may irritate the uterus lining, or from the hormonal drugs, but it can also be implantation spotting that happens when the embryo burrows into the lining of your uterus and implants itself to begin growing. You can do a pregnancy test on day fourteen and let us know the results. You can test from day eleven, but we recommend you wait. Do you have any questions?'

I had a million questions. Would it work? Would I have twins? Would they be healthy? Was all spotting good? What if I didn't have spotting – did that mean it wasn't working? How can I wait two weeks to find out? But they weren't questions she could answer. Now it was a waiting game.

The Two-Week Wait

Fourteen Days. Two weeks. 336 hours. 20,160 minutes. 1,209, 600 seconds.

Arghhhhhhhhhhhhhhhh!

It's a lifetime. Infertility hell. It's how long I wished the time was when we were having that fab holiday in Thailand three years ago, but it seemed to zoom past in a flash. Now it was the opposite. I wanted to blink and it would be over, but it was there, looming on forever in the distance. Why was it when you wanted the time to go quickly it never did? A letter by snail mail used to take seven days to arrive and now it's an email that takes a second to be delivered. A boat journey to Australia used to take six weeks. Now, it's a twenty-four hour flight away. So why did it take two sodding weeks to find out if you were pregnant?

I'd already had so many two-week waits, wondering if this would be the month I'd get pregnant, but this, by far, was the most important one.

I decided to stay in bed for two days, just to be on the safe side. I mean, what if the embryos accidentally fell out while I was walking around? I couldn't take the risk.

I was so in tune with my body it was like I'd put myself under a magnifying glass. Was that cramping I just felt or wind? What was that twinge? I need a wee again. Hang on a sec…didn't I just go a minute ago? Frequent urination was a sign of pregnancy – it must be working! God, my boobs are sore. Yep, another sure sign. And they've grown. Note to self: If I start spotting, it must be implantation spotting and must definitely *not* be confused with my period.

I promised myself I wasn't going to go on the internet and

219

start checking out symptoms of pregnancy again. In fact, I wouldn't go on it at all. I would ban myself from it completely. It had been one of my best friends in my quest to get pregnant but it could also be my enemy.

I didn't last long. Four hours, eight wees, and a twinge later, I was on my laptop in bed, where I discovered stories of women following a diet high in yams prior to embryo transfer, because apparently there was a tribe of African women who were the most fertile in the world who ate a diet high in yams. It was the same tribe that drank the wee. Weird. Then there was another story about Cold Uterus Syndrome. Apparently, if you had cold feet it meant your uterus was cold, which equalled poor blood flow to the embryos and lack of nutrition, so hundreds of women were walking around twenty-four hours a day with thick socks on to counteract it.

What? Why wasn't I told this? Why didn't Dr Swanson insist I eat lots of yams and wear socks? Could we even get yams here? I'd never seen them in the supermarket. And did a sweet potato count as the same thing? Another note to self: send Karl out for a kilo of sweet potatoes when he gets home.

For the first few days, I stared at the two pictures of my embryos, scrutinizing them. If I held them in a particular light, could I see what sex they were? Wait, was one of the two fuzzy specks on the ultrasound picture actually smiling at me? Two amazing, miracle little specks. Six cells and four cells. If I added that up together it made ten cells, which meant they were perfectly developed, didn't it? I felt so proud of myself. I felt happy. I'd come this far and it would work. Definitely, positively, absolutely would work.

I meditated in bed and used Suzanne's visualization techniques. I saw my embryos burrowing in, growing stronger by the second. I told myself over and over again that they would strengthen into healthy babies. I begged Zelda to make it happen.

On the third day, I got out of bed and pottered around the

house. I spoke to Amelia, Poppy, and Suzanne on the phone, who were there to give me support. Poppy didn't even mind me ringing her at all hours to talk about this twinge or that little spot of blood I'd discovered. It was a good sign to have those cramps, wasn't it? The doctor had said it could be the embryos burrowing in. Were the cramps I was getting implantation cramps? Yes, they must be. Only another infertile woman could talk for two hours about cramps. I phoned Kerry to talk about Elise, hoping that her baby vibes would transfer down the phone to my uterus. I wore two pairs of socks at all times.

On day four, I had some clients booked in, which I was hoping would take my mind off thinking, but it didn't. Everyone was asking me how things were going, and it was all I wanted to talk about, and all I could think about. I asked Karl to reassure me that if I hadn't eaten millions of yams or drunk wee before the IVF it would still work. He affirmed that not only had I been eating a perfectly healthy diet all this time, but that my uterus was a warm and cosy place to be, with or without socks. I promised myself (another one!) that I wouldn't do a pregnancy test until at least day fourteen.

On day five, I visited Suzanne for crystal healing. She let me ramble on excitedly about everything. How I was craving pickles, how my boobs were sore, how my jeans didn't fit me like they did the day before. That could only mean one thing, couldn't it? On the way home, a butterfly landed on me and I just knew it was a sign from Zelda telling me that my embryos were happy and healthy.

On day six, I was on the internet again. I couldn't help myself. Most of the internet searches for fertility stories had to do with pregnancy symptoms: *Cramping after IVF treatment. Do sore breasts after IVF equal pregnancy? Is spotting after IVF normal? Can wearing socks improve uterus nutrition for embryos?*

What if I did a pregnancy test now? Would it show up? There was one woman on Fertility Friends who tested on day six and got a positive reading. Should I do it, too? If I tested now and it was negative that meant it still wouldn't be final. If it was negative, I'd still have a chance at being pregnant. I mean, I was sure I *was* pregnant, so really it was just a formality. But deep down, even though I was sure, I had a teensy weensy part of my brain in doubt. Did I want the fantasy of finally being pregnant to end?

On day seven, my boobs were so sore I couldn't sleep on my front anymore. That had to be a good sign. I couldn't stand it anymore. I cracked and did a pregnancy test. It was negative. Even though I knew it was way too soon, part of me told me it was over. I wasn't pregnant. But then the other part of me shouted in my head: *You had cramps. You had spotting. It was definitely implantation spotting. They're still there, burrowing away in your very warm uterus. It's too soon to test.* I cried for the first time. Then I went back on the Internet and pored over articles, only reading the ones that confirmed what I was praying was true. It was definitely too early to get a positive result. It wasn't over yet. Karl told me off for testing too early, and I asked him to hide all the pregnancy tests I'd amassed.

On day eight, I was feeling restless. I couldn't sit down, I couldn't stand still, I was spacey, I couldn't sleep. My brain felt sluggish, like I'd turned into a slow-worm overnight. I needed to know. I rummaged around in the house to try and find where Karl had hidden the tests. I couldn't find them so I went out and bought one, and tested again. I know, I know, but all the waiting was frying my brain. It was negative. I rang all my friends, wanting reassurance that it was still too early.

On day nine, I vowed not to go on the Internet or test again. This time I managed it, although the what ifs were creeping in big time. What if it this treatment failed? Should we try again? Do I want to try again? What if we go to Australia? What if it didn't work out when we got there? What if I really was crazy for thinking about travelling? Then I pushed all the negative thoughts to the back of my head and replaced them with happy, positive ones. I didn't want to obsess about it. I was sick to death of obsessing.

I went for a long walk with Karl, who tried to take my mind off things by cracking jokes. We watched DVDs. Anything not to try and think. I even cleaned out my cupboards, believing that the sudden urge was my body's way of telling me to do the nesting thing.

On day ten, I was having a breathing exercise and meditation-fest. Suzanne came to the house and did them with me before giving me a crystal healing session. It relaxed me for about five minutes, until the pull of the pregnancy tests were getting too much for me to cope with. Dr Swanson said I could test tomorrow but it was better to wait for day fourteen. Should I test? No. I should wait. Could I wait, though? That was the question. Yes, of course I could. It wasn't like I was impatient or anything. Much.

On day eleven, I woke up with severe cramps. I lay in the darkness, willing them to go away. After an hour, they were still there so I went to the bathroom to check for blood.

I wiped myself.

No blood.

Phew!

But even though there was no blood I felt like I wasn't pregnant. Then I pushed the thought away. If I didn't think it or say it out loud then it wouldn't become a reality. Technically, I could do the test now and find out. That was what Dr Swanson had said, but should I wait? Maybe the cramps didn't mean anything. Maybe they were normal. I tortured myself in the darkness, wondering what to do. I woke Karl and asked his opinion. He said I should wait, so he held me tight in the darkness until the morning. Then I was back on the Internet, searching for signs of hope.

No, cramps didn't always mean you weren't pregnant. Yes, it could still have worked.

Right. OK. Take a deep breath. Relax.

Relax? Yeah, right!

On day twelve, I had a monster headache but I wouldn't

223

take anything for it. No drugs were passing my lips until I knew the truth. I don't know how I got through the day without turning into a complete basket case, but somehow I did. I tried to push all thoughts of it out of my head. And it worked, too. For about five seconds.

On day thirteen, I couldn't wait any longer. I'd bought a special digital thermometer for the occasion because I couldn't be messing around looking for two lines on the other ones. I wanted it spelled out to me in black and white "Pregnant." My plan was to wake up at seven and take the test. When I got the positive result, I'd rush off to the supermarket and buy a congratulations on being a dad card for Karl. Then I'd scrawl in it in baby handwriting, as if it were from our little beans to their daddy.

Instead, I woke up at five a.m. and crept into the bathroom.

I peed on the test stick.

I waited the two agonizing minutes.

I looked at the digital readout.

Not Pregnant.

I couldn't cry straight away. I was in shock.

It had failed. I had failed. I had failed him.

I didn't want to believe it, but as I stared at the readout, I had to believe it. It was there, shouting at me. Screaming at me in the silence. But then a thought wormed its way into my brain. Were the digital tests not as sensitive as the ones with lines? I was sure I'd read that somewhere during my many hours on the Internet. Maybe I should try the other ones.

I'd found Karl's secret stash of pregnancy tests the day before so I pulled all twelve out and tried again.

Test one: Negative.

Test two: Negative.

Test three: Negative.

Test four: Negative.

I knew I should've given up then but I used all twelve. They were all the same.

I went into the bedroom to wake up Karl. I didn't want to

cry alone, and he was the only other person in the world who wanted it more than me.

'I'm not pregnant,' my voice came out husky in the darkness, like it belonged to someone else.

The look on his face broke my heart into a thousand pieces. 'Are you sure? It's only day thirteen. Maybe it's too early.'

I shook my head. 'The tests can read the results two days before you're due. Dr Swanson said I could test from day eleven. There is no baby. Our beautiful, miracle embryos died.'

And as he reached out to me and pulled me into his arms on the bed I let out a strangled yell of hurt and anger so loud it sounded like a wounded animal.

Then I cried. I cried like I'd never done before. I cried so hard I was silent. I pressed my hands hard against my eyes, trying to push the tears back inside me. Trying to push the hurt back inside. And as he buried his face into my neck, I felt his own hot tears on my skin.

We both knew it was over.

Goodbye

My period arrived with a vengeance the next day, dashing any small hope I had that all the tests were wrong. I felt angry. Why give us a glimmer of hope only to snatch it away again? I wanted to blame someone. The doctors, the nurses, Karl, Zelda, myself, anyone. Was it something I'd done? Was it because I preferred lie-ins instead of exercise in my twenties? Was it because I ate too much junk food when I was younger? Drank too much alcohol? Had too many late nights? Was it something in my genes? Would I have got pregnant if I'd started trying earlier? Or had the doctors messed up the embryo transfer somehow?

But I knew no one was to blame. It just happened.

I felt gut-wrenching sadness that was like physical pain. I was left with joylessness and hopelessness. I hated myself and I hated the world. My heart was broken. How was I going to face tomorrow? Or the next day? Or the day after that? Our final chance at conceiving had just vanished, along with my fantasy of being pregnant. Now what?

I couldn't talk to anyone, not even Karl. For the first two days, I lay on the sofa in the lounge with the TV on. I stared at it so I wouldn't have to think. David Attenborough was having a Blue Planet Special weekend on National Geographic channel. For forty-eight hours, I lay in the same position watching whales and dolphins and sharks and seals. Somehow, his soft voice was really soothing and the animal noises seemed to comfort me. Occasionally, I'd doze off, only to be woken by horrible dreams of dying embryos that looked like plump grapes, then shrivelled into raisins before my eyes. I'd scream and Karl would come running downstairs to rock me until I fell asleep again.

After the weekend, Karl went back to work. He said he needed to get his mind off it. I knew by his actions that he was devastated in a thousand ways, and he looked at me like he was worried to death about whether I would cope with this, but I couldn't deal with how he felt. I could only deal with my feelings.

Karl had cancelled my clients, and I ignored the phone that rang constantly and the knocks on the door. I wanted to stay in a cocoon for the rest of my life, not thinking or feeling anything.

I wandered around the house aimlessly, feeling brittle, like I could shatter into shreds at any second. I stared at our embryo pictures for hours. I saw the fertility drugs in the bathroom and kitchen, thinking how much better life was before I found out. How could I ever go back to the way things were? I couldn't.

After all the tests, drugs, needles, scans, worry, eggs being sucked out, eggs being pushed in, and interminable waiting, I was left with nothing except disappointment and loss.

This went on for two weeks. I lost weight, I had dark circles under my eyes; no one could reach me. Everything was a constant reminder: as I packed away all the IVF drugs; when I took down the post-it notes with pregnancy mantras; when I went to the shops to buy food in a daze and accidentally found myself in the baby aisle; when I turned on the TV and saw adverts for nappies. It was my birthday in four days but I didn't feel like celebrating. I felt like I was imploding into a huge pit of grief. I wanted attention and comforting hugs from Karl, but at the same time, I wanted to be alone.

Suzanne came round to visit me and stood on the doorstep, refusing to leave until I let her in. When I opened the door she didn't need to say anything, she just hugged me. I couldn't cry anymore. I didn't have any tears left.

'Karl phoned me,' she said. 'He's worried about you.'

'I know he is. I'm worried about me.'

227

'That's why I'm here. I want to help,' she said as we went inside, her arm firmly around my shoulder.

'I don't want to talk about it. It's still too raw,' I said.

'OK, I'll talk and you listen. If I can give you something positive to clutch onto, then I'll feel like I've been useful.' She held my shoulders and looked into my eyes with so much concentration it was as if she could read my soul. 'Is that OK?'

I nodded.

'This grief you're feeling is a part of the healing process, but you have to be careful it doesn't consume you. It will get easier. Healing takes time, and often, growth and wisdom follow loss.'

I snorted. I didn't want to hear that.

'It's true. After everything you've put your body and mind through, it's natural to feel like this. And just like you did the fertility treatment, now you have to treat yourself to get well.' She paused, making sure she had my full attention. 'It's the death of a dream, but it's not death. You and Karl will still go on. There's plenty of living to be done.'

I thought about that for a moment and knew she was right. I'd hit the bottom and now I had to find a way to stagger to my feet again. Life would go on, and I had to find a way to live again.

'You said before you wouldn't be able to go back to the old you, and that's true,' she said. 'You've been on an incredible journey, and there's no way you can be the same as you were before all this started. But now you have to look to the future. You need to celebrate what you already have. Instead of concentrating on all the things that have gone wrong, concentrate on what has gone right. Put up a picture of you and Karl and remind yourself every day what you're grateful for. Before you get out of bed in the morning, tell yourself there are so many brand new possibilities for you today. You're healthy, you have each other, your life can go anywhere from here. Don't think about where you wanted things to go, think about where they *will* go from here.'

228

I nodded glumly, taking in what she was saying.

'Should you sacrifice living for something you've never had?' she asked me, studying my face. 'Destroy your own life so you can try and create another?'

'No,' I admitted. And I knew she was absolutely right. My guru always seemed to say exactly the right things.

Karl and I had got through this together. He'd put up with me turning into a complete psycho for two years. How many men would do that? We'd survived it. We would survive it. I was grateful to have the man I loved more than anything in the world standing by my side. If we couldn't have a family, we would still have each other. I was blessed with a man who loved me back. A man who was in it for the long haul. We'd been through the good times and survived the rough times. We could do it again. Karl was still there, standing tall for me. And in some ways I felt our relationship would be even stronger now after all that we'd gone through.

I vowed there and then that I would never hope to get pregnant again. I know hope is a wonderful thing, but sometimes you have to let it go. I couldn't spend the next unknown amount of years hoping month upon month that I'd get lucky. I was fed up with being a mean, depressed, emotional car crash. I desperately wanted and needed to have a child with Karl but it wouldn't happen. It obviously wasn't meant to happen. So that just meant there was something else for us. Would that something be Australia? I'd spent the last two years being upset, unhappy, angry, frustrated, bitchy, tearful, crazy, instead of the old normal me who had a great social life, enjoyed her job, kicked back and relaxed. I didn't want to be the person I'd become anymore. It was taking over our lives. I knew I couldn't go on like this, freewheeling out of control both mentally and physically. I couldn't put myself through IVF again. I couldn't do it to my body, my mind, or our marriage. Every brand new day there was a new choice, a new direction to take. That's what I had to think about now. Instead of being in limbo agony, I had to choose to be free again.

I poured my heart out to Suzanne, telling her about the plans I'd been thinking about if things didn't work out.

'Well, that certainly is drastic.' Suzanne smiled at me for the first time that day. 'I think it takes a very strong and brave person to give up on their hopes and dreams and start a new chapter.'

'I need to do something drastic. That's the whole point.' I shrugged. 'I'm now closer to forty than thirty and my life is running away from me. What have I got to show for it? You said that there are so many new possibilities out there...I think this is one of them.'

'Change can be such a good thing if it gives you the strength to carry on and empowers you. I think you should discuss it with Karl. It's a fantastic idea.' Her eyes lit up. 'Although I'll miss you. I think we've become good friends.'

I threw my arms around her. 'You're my guru, Suzanne. You've kept me sane. I don't know how I would've got through all this stuff without you.'

She patted my back and laughed softly. 'I told you, Gina, *you're* the guru.'

When she left I rushed down the shops to buy a red balloon. It had to be red to symbolize love. It was time to say an official goodbye to my embryos and my dream.

I went out into the garden where it had all begun two years ago with the vision of a baby. Now I was going to put it to rest. I drew a heart on the balloon and wrote one word on it: *Goodbye*. Then I thought that was a bit short so I added more hearts and some kisses.

I took a deep breath and looked up at the clouds, pressing the balloon close to my heart. I closed my eyes. Then I let the balloon float up into the sky, just like I'd done all those months ago with the imaginary balloon I'd sent to Zelda, feeling that I'd come full circle. All my hopes, my fears, my neurotic behaviour, my dreams of being a parent – now was the time to let it all go.

I watched it until it became a speck in the distance. It

wasn't until it had completely disappeared from view that I turned and walked back into the house.

I went upstairs, flicked through our wedding albums and chose a picture of Karl and me staring into each other's eyes with an ecstatic grin. I put it in a silver photo frame by my bed and traced his face with my fingertip.

Now it was time for a new life. I was getting out of the baby trap.

One Day at a Time

The next day, I woke up feeling lighter and freer than I had in months. The first thought I had wasn't what day is it in my cycle, or which test or hormone drug should I be taking today. It was a brand new start, and I had a great feeling about it.

I slid out of bed without waking Karl and padded downstairs to make breakfast – the first meal I'd made in ages. Instead of having an empty pit in my stomach, I felt ravenous. I could eat anything I wanted from now on. I could get pissed on red wine again. My life wouldn't be ruled by calendars anymore. We could have fun doing things we enjoyed together, instead of getting stressed and fighting. I would be witty again and funny and make Karl laugh like I used to.

Bacon and eggs. Yep, that's what I wanted. Greasy bacon and eggs, mushrooms, tomatoes, and toast. I wasn't going to blow all my healthy eating habits, but I was going to treat us to a fab fry-up to celebrate new beginnings. No more anxiety or stress about trying to get pregnant. No more doctors or hospital visits. No more intolerable waiting. I was going to live in the moment.

I rushed out of the house to the corner shop and came back with the makings of a sumptuous feast.

When Karl stumbled downstairs, he studied me carefully, unsure what mood I'd be in. 'Are you OK?' He leaned on the doorway, with wary eyes, like maybe I'd completely tipped over the edge and cooking a fry-up was the first sign of a nervous breakdown.

'I'm fine!' I beamed back at him, brimming with

confidence as I cracked a couple of eggs into the frying pan.

He walked up behind me and put his arms around my waist, resting his head on my shoulders. 'It's good to have you back.'

I turned to face him and looped my arms around his neck. 'It's good to be back.' I nuzzled into him. 'I'm sorry I've been a nightmare.'

'You don't have to apologize. It's hard. We're both grieving.'

'I know,' I said, determined not to cry.

'We'll get though it. One day at a time, it will get easier.' His face radiated with love.

Australia Here We Come

For the next few days, I buried myself in work and the Internet, searching sites about Australia. Anything to stop me thinking. Even though I'd said goodbye to my hopes and dreams, I was still going through the grieving process, and I knew the only thing that would heal it was time. A cliché, I know, but I really believed it. How would I feel six months from now? A year? It would get easier with every day, but I wanted to push the unhappy thoughts to the back of my head and concentrate on something else. I knew it would take a long time to get to a place where I was comfortable with the realization I'd never be a mother, but I had to start living again.

As I went through the websites, I realized I didn't want to plan anything. I was sick of planning. I'd been planning everything in my life around my cycle, my temperature, my hormone treatments, and my egg white. Now was the time to be unpredictable, spontaneous. The way I saw it, all we really needed to do was rent out the house, get our visa and flight tickets, and go. I wanted an adventure, where I didn't know what was going to happen the next day, or the next. I wanted excitement. I wanted to experience wonderful new possibilities every day.

Every time Karl came in when I was on the Internet I'd close the tab and pretend I was looking at something else. I'd decided to wait until my birthday to bring up my plans with him since I figured how could he refuse me on my birthday? Hey, you can't blame a girl for being sneaky!

The night before I turned thirty-five, Amelia, Dan, Kerry, and Mark came round bearing bottles of wine and pressies.

234

'Omigod!' I squealed. 'This is the first glass of wine I've had in soooo long. It's so yum.' I savoured my first mouthful, knowing I'd probably be tipsy before I'd finished it.

'Well, it gets better,' Kerry said, handing me the biggest box of chocolates I'd ever seen in my life.

'Aw.' I licked my lips, grinning. 'I'm not sharing these with anyone.'

Amelia cornered me in the kitchen later on while the others were laughing and joking in the lounge. 'Are you OK? We've all been worried about you.'

I always hated it when people asked you if you were OK. It was usually my cue to burst into tears. But I was sick of crying. 'I will be. Eventually.'

She gave me a hug, sensing I didn't want to talk about anything.

'I'm going to ask Karl about Australia tomorrow,' I said. 'Wish me luck.'

Amelia's eyes widened. 'So you really want to do it?'

'I feel like it's something I have to do to get myself back. To get us back again. All this stuff really takes it out of you.'

'If you go, what am I going to do without you?' This time it was Amelia's turn to cry instead of mine. Her eyes glistened in the kitchen light. 'I'll miss you so much. We all will.'

'Oh, don't cry. I'm going to miss you guys loads, too.' I grabbed her hand. 'I don't know if it's going to happen for real yet. It depends on what Karl thinks, but if we go, it probably won't be forever. We'll still see each other. Don't worry, you can't get rid of me that easily. You'll get loads of emails from me, and phone calls.'

She sniffed, smiling at me. 'You'd better.' She poked me in the ribs. 'So, what's Karl got planned for tomorrow, then?'

'I don't know. He said it was a big surprise.'

'Oooh, interesting.' She raised an eyebrow.

'Hmm. I'm not sure that surprises are good when you're

235

nearly forty, they might induce heart attacks, strokes, and possible sudden bowel movements.'

She snorted. 'You're not nearly forty!'

'Well, thirty-five is closer to forty than thirty.'

'Maybe you're having a midlife crisis,' she giggled.

'Maybe I am.'

Birthday Surprise!

Birthday. Birth Day. A day of life. It was the day I was brought into the world, and now I knew my child would never have a birthday. But instead of dwelling on morbid thoughts, I looked at the picture of Karl and me on our wedding day.

Celebrate what you have. Don't grieve for what you never had. Don't sacrifice living.

I could hear Karl bashing around downstairs making me breakfast in bed, which would probably be a bowl of organic porridge.

'Da da,' he said five minutes later as he swung into the bedroom balancing a tray.

I pushed the duvet back and sat up. 'Wow.' I looked at a bowl of fresh fruit salad, topped with kiwi and blueberries, and a single red rose stuffed into a pint glass. 'What an effort you've gone to,' I exclaimed.

'You thought it would be porridge, didn't you?' He smirked at me.

'No!' I grinned, stroking his arm. 'It's lovely.' I took a mouthful. OK, so I actually hated blueberries, but it was the thought that counted.

'Wait there, I'm going to get your pressie.' He stomped back downstairs and returned a few minutes later.

'Ooh, I wonder what this can be.' I took the present from his outstretched hand and unwrapped it. 'Ah, perfume. What a nice surprise, thanks.' I smirked at him. 'So you're not having a secret affair with Britney, then?

'Well, actually I am, but seeing as she's out of town today I thought I'd take my gorgeous wife out for a birthday lunch

237

instead.' He kissed me softly on the cheek and perched on the edge of the bed, looking very proud of himself. 'And actually, that's not the surprise. You'll have to wait until later to find out.' He glanced at his watch. 'I've got that important breakfast meeting with Clive, so I'll be back a bit later.'

'When was the last time we went out for lunch?' I said wistfully.

'Too long ago.'

I reached up and traced his cheek with my fingertip. 'What did I do to deserve you?'

He took hold of my fingers and slid them through his, pressing them against his cheek. 'Despite all the stress we've been through in the last couple of years, I love you more today than I did before. I'm so proud of you. The way you go for what you want. The way you never give up on things. You're an amazing woman.'

Now that did bring tears to my eyes again. What was wrong with me? I was turning into a blubber machine. 'I've been a horrible nightmare!'

He chuckled. 'Well, yes, that, too, but that's understandable.'

'Well, I...I need to talk to you about something, actually.'

He pressed a finger to my lips. 'I need to talk to you, too, but I have to go. We'll do it at lunch.' He kissed me goodbye, and I made sure I ate every last blueberry.

We went to a quiet little country pub with wooden beams, low ceilings, and little snug areas to sit. It was just right.

I shrugged off my coat and rubbed my hands together in front of the log fire crackling away next to our table. 'We really should to do this more often.'

'From now on, we will.' Karl ginned and studied his menu. 'What are you having?'

My eyes wandered to the specials board. 'Mmm, they've got mussels in garlic sauce. That's what I'm having.'

'Are they organic?' He raised an enquiring eyebrow.

'Listen…I've been thinking…' I changed the subject.

'Oh no, I hate it when you think,' he butted in, chuckling.

'Ha ha. Do you want to hear it or not?' I gazed at him over the rim of my wine glass.

'Let me go and order first and then tell me.' He took himself and his menu off to the bar.

I picked at my thumbnail, waiting for him to return.

'Right. What were you thinking?' He sat down and looked at me with interest.

'Well, lately I think we've been stuck in a rut. I feel like I've been on this big stressed-out rollercoaster for years over this fertility stuff, and it just seems like we're drifting apart because of it. We both haven't been happy lately, and I need to find something else to concentrate on now that…'

He nodded. 'I know.'

'And…'

He reached out and put his hand in mine. 'And, what?'

'And we need to find *each other* again. I'm bored with our life. I've been unsociable, ratty, grumpy, upset. I want to get the old me back, but at the same time I can't go back to the old me.' I leaned forward and tried to gauge what he was thinking. 'I need to find myself again.'

He looked shocked. 'Are you bored with me?' He looked around the room to see if anyone was listening.

'No!' I replied instantly. 'No, I just…I just want something more out of life if I can't have a baby. I've finally got to the point where enough is enough.' I gripped his hand. 'I want to–'

'Oh, my God! Are you trying to say you want to split up?' he whispered. 'I mean, I know I probably haven't been as sensitive and supportive about this whole business as I should have been. I know you've been really down about it, but…' He ran a hand through his hair, looking worried.

'No,' I insisted. 'I don't want to split up,' I whispered back. 'I want to travel round Australia. With you.'

'You had me worried there for a minute.' He reached for my hand and smiled. 'And it's so strange because I've been sort of thinking about the same thing myself. You do need something else to focus on. But I was thinking more about getting a tortoise.'

'A tortoise!' I blustered.

He frowned. 'What's wrong with that?'

'I'm afraid a tortoise just isn't going to do it for me. I have to do something extreme. I need an adventure. Something spontaneous where we can have fun and experience possibilities we didn't even know about. I've been researching it on the Internet. We could rent out the house to pay for it, get a couple of flights, and just go where the mood takes us. No pressure. No calendars to follow. Get our life back somewhere where there are no reminders about babies.' I paused, glancing down at my fingernail that I'd chewed to oblivion. 'It just feels like the right thing to do. It feels like I need to do it. We need to do it. I want to live in the moment again and appreciate what we have.'

'Oh.' He looked gobsmacked. 'Wow. That's *definitely* extreme,' he finally said.

'Not really.' I shook my head.

Then he started laughing, eyeing me with a twinkle.

'What?' I said. 'Why are you laughing?'

'Do you really think I didn't know what you were up to? Every time I walked in the room and you were on the Internet, you'd pretend you were looking at something else.'

'What do you mean?'

'One day I came in and you closed down a tab, and when I looked over your shoulder you were staring, seemingly fascinated by a website about photocopiers.'

I sat back, trying to remember. 'Was I?'

He nodded. 'And Amelia told Dan, who didn't know it was a secret, and he told me about what you wanted to do.'

I drained the last of my fruity red wine for courage and swallowed. 'So, what do you think? I know you'd have to give up your job, and I know they've been pushing you hard lately about sales figures and you've been getting pissed off with it, anyway, so maybe this is the perfect time for a career change. And if we really liked it out there, maybe we could stay. Get a working visa. Maybe you'd end up with an even better job. Apparently, they've got a lack of telecommunications bods out there. And–'

He put his hand up to silence my babbling. Then he reached for his pint of beer and took a long, slow sip.

Oh, shit. He was going to say no. He was going to tell me he hated that idea. That I was being ridiculous. Impulsive. That all the hormone drugs had fried my brain. And what if he did say no? This was something I really needed to do. Would we split up because he didn't want to come with me?

He put his drink down and reached into his jacket pocket.

I peered over, trying to get a glimpse at what he was doing.

Then he handed me two passports.

I took them, my eyebrows questioning his face.

He nodded at the passports. 'Look inside.'

I opened them up and flicked through them. Inside were twelve month visas for us to visit Australia.

My jaw pinged open. It didn't quite hit the floor, but it was close. 'Wow!'

'The tortoise was just a wind up to throw you off the scent.' He threw his head back and roared with laughter, then clutched his chest and doubled up, howling. Then he nodded at the passports. 'That's your birthday surprise. I think it's a great idea. It could be just what we need after everything that's happened. I don't relish the thought of staying here when I'd just be reminded about the fact I can't be a dad every day. We do need a fresh start somewhere totally different.'

I jumped up and launched myself onto his lap, much to the amusement of the waitress, who was bringing over our food. 'We're going to Australia! We're going to Australia,' I squealed. As the waitress put the plates on the table I told her, 'We're going to Australia!'

She looked at me like I was slightly nuts and nodded. 'Sounds wonderful.'

'Can we have a bottle of red wine, please?' Karl asked her.

'Would you like the house red or something else?' She tilted her head.

Karl looked a me. 'Actually, make it a bottle of Moët champagne. This is a celebration, after all.'

'So…' I jumped off his lap and sat down, picking at my food, 'where shall we fly to? Sydney, Adelaide, Perth?' I waved my fork around with animation.

Karl tucked into his steak. 'Sydney sounds good.'

'I can ring the estate agent and get them round so we can rent out the house.' I forked a soft mussel into my mouth.

'My breakfast meeting this morning with Clive was about handing in my notice.' He put his fork down and finished off his beer.

'Oh!' I looked up. 'Well, you don't mess around, either. What did he say?'

'He doesn't want me to go. He offered me a huge package to stay, actually.' He paused for a minute to take a bite of steak. 'And *then* he tells me that they're looking into setting up a sister company in Australia next year, and would I go over and head up the new division in Sydney,' he said, looking pretty pleased with himself. 'That would give us plenty of time to travel around and do exactly what we want before we have to get back into a routine again.'

My hands flew to my mouth. 'Agh! Really? That's fantastic. I mean, I knew they were thinking about expanding to America, but Australia, too? Wow!' I thought about what Suzanne had said about projecting stuff out to the Universe and trusting that what you want will happen. Maybe Zelda had got her wires crossed, and instead of picking up my messages about babies, she was giving me the opportunity of Australia instead. Didn't Suzanne say if it's meant to be, it will happen? So my purpose in life wasn't to be a mother. Instead, it was something beckoning me in Australia. All the pieces were beginning to fit together so perfectly it had to be right.

'Yep. It is, isn't it? He looked pretty pleased with himself as the waitress brought over the champagne.

'Would you like me to open it, or do you want to do the honours?' She looked at Karl.

Karl reached for the bottle. 'I'll do it.' He popped the cork perfectly, without spilling a drop, and poured out two glasses for us. He passed one to me and held his up in front of him. 'To new beginnings.' He gazed at me intently.

'To new beginnings.' I clinked his glass with mine, falling in love with him all over again for the second time that day.

We chatted excitedly over more champers about all the places we could visit and adventures we could have. For the first time in what felt like a lifetime, I savoured the feeling of being relaxed and happy. This is what living in the moment was all about. As we stood up to leave, Karl whispered in my ear. 'We haven't made love in a long time.'

I giggled, the champers had gone to my head ages ago. 'Huh? We've had so much sex I'm surprised you haven't had to have a replacement willy,' I whispered back, grabbing onto his shoulder to stop me swaying.

'Exactly. We've been having sex. We haven't been making love.'

I nuzzled into his neck. 'So what are we waiting for? Let's go home and make love.'

As soon as we got home, our clothes were off and we were in the bedroom, but this time we were enjoying exploring each other's bodies again as if it were the first time. There were no rushed moves to just get it over with. No contortionist positions. No invasive thoughts, wondering if this would be the time I got pregnant. Just our bodies in tune with each other as we moved to our own rhythm, staring in each other's eyes, with the sound of the rain outside, delicately tapping on the window.

Thanks Zelda!

The next four weeks flew by in a daze. I didn't have time to stop and think about whether we were crazy for doing this, or whether things would work out. There was so much to organize to keep me occupied. A guy who Karl worked with wanted to rent our house fully furnished, so all we needed to do was store our personal belongings. We'd bought our one-way tickets to Sydney, and we had a hotel booked for just two nights. Whatever happened after that was anybody's guess. I figured Zelda would send me a sign, anyway.

As I boxed up the last of our belongings, I looked around the house that had been my home for five years, but I didn't feel sad. I felt excited. Yes, I was also going to miss everyone like crazy, but I knew in my heart we were doing the right thing.

Karl came home from work as I was in the bathroom, going through a cupboard that hadn't been cleared out in a long time so I could get rid of all the junk before we rented the house. I pulled out a stray pregnancy test that had fallen to the back.

'Well, I won't need that anymore,' I said, staring at it. And for once, I didn't have a gut-wrenching pain in me. Don't get me wrong, I was sad. I did have a hole there, but it was getting easier to deal with. I wasn't going to let it consume me anymore. Every second of every day, time was healing my ache.

'I'll throw it away, shall I?' Karl said, rubbing my shoulder.

'Yep. Throw it...' And then I had a weird thought. Hang on a sec, when was my last period? With all that had been going on I'd completely forgotten about it. I tilted my head, tapping my lips. I hadn't had one since after the IVF, which was seven weeks before.

'What?' Karl said.

I swung around to face him. 'I haven't had my period.'

'Maybe the IVF messed up your cycle, and you're going to be late this month.'

I nodded, not daring to even think of the other possibility. 'You're right. Throw it.' I handed it to him and he wandered off downstairs to chuck it away.

'Wait!' I called over the banister to him. 'Maybe I should use it.'

His face crumpled. 'Gina…you're probably just late.'

'I know, I know, but…what if?'

'Are you sure you want to do this?' The pained expression on his face told me he knew it would only be a setback for me if it was negative.

No, I wasn't sure. I hadn't felt sick. My boobs weren't aching. I poked them, just in case. Nope, definitely not sore. I would only be torturing myself but…what if I was?

'I'm sure.' I nodded, biting my lip.

He walked back upstairs and handed it over, then he backed out the door and wandered into the bedroom. 'I can't look.'

I took it with shaky hands, unpeeling the wrapper quickly before I could change my mind. This was a ridiculous idea. Of course I wasn't pregnant.

You're just late, that's all. You're going to Australia, you can't be pregnant, I thought as I peed on the gazillionth test of my life.

I placed the stick on the edge of the bath, knowing it was going to be negative.

You're just using up the last one. Might as well use it, rather than chuck it away. A final farewell to all things pregnancy related.

I carried on clearing out the cupboard so I wouldn't look at it. Old, crusty makeup, a very tattered face cloth, a nailbrush

245

with half the bristles missing. Why had I kept this stuff?

As I leaned back to put them in a pile on the floor my gaze caught the result box on the test.

'Agh!' I croaked, suddenly losing the use of my legs and dropping to the floor in a crumpled heap.

'Oh, God,' Karl's voice drifted from the bedroom. 'I knew you shouldn't have done it. 'Don't worry, babe. We're going to Australia. New beginnings, remember? You just have to concentrate on that.' He appeared at the bathroom door.

I waved the stick around, my mouth flapping open and closed like a goldfish.

'We'll get through this.' He sat on the floor next to me.

'Look!' I shoved the stick in his face.

Two lines. Two strong blue lines.

I was pregnant.

Karl looked from the test to me, and back to the test again. 'Does that really mean what I think it means?'

I nodded, momentarily losing my power of speech.

He pulled me up, jumping up and down with me. 'I'm going to be a dad!'

I threw my arms around his neck. 'I'm going to be a mum!' I grinned so wide I was surprised my teeth didn't fall out.

'Wow!'

'Double wow!'

'This is unbelievable,' he said, then suddenly stopped jumping. 'What about Australia?'

'Yes! What about Australia?' I thought about it for a minute, my mind a whirlwind of excitement. 'I think we should still go. Why not take each day as it comes for a while? We can still travel round for a few months and just see what happens. I think living in the moment will be calming for the baby.' I rubbed my stomach, wondering if he or she could hear us. 'The way I see it, we've got two choices. We can go to Oz like we planned, and if it's meant to be, you'll head up Carl's new company there after we've had a fabulous time travelling. If it's not meant to be, then we will have had the best extended holiday of our lives, and it'll give us the chance to relax after the last couple of stressful years. What do you think?'

He put his hand next to mine on my stomach, gazing with awe at the little life it contained inside. 'What do you think, Cecil? Shall we go to Australia and see where life takes us?' He looked into my eyes, grinning. 'You decide.'

'Let's go and live in the moment.'

He picked me up and swung me around with joy. 'New beginnings and adventures in Australia, it is, then.'

I threw my head back to the ceiling and whispered, 'Thank you, Zelda.'

'Who's Zelda?'

I grinned. 'It's a long story.'

The End

A note from the author:

I'd like to say a big thanks for buying The Baby Trap. Even though it's fiction, this story is based on a lot of my own experiences with infertility. Hubby and I tried for five years to have a baby and endured two rounds of IVF without success. It took a really long time for me to get to a place where I was OK with knowing I'd never get pregnant. Eventually, I was lucky enough to find a new direction in my life that gave me something else to think about, and that was writing. Now my books are my babies (oh, and my eight rescue cats!)

For anyone going through struggles to achieve their dreams in life (and that goes for anything, not just infertility), I'm wishing you all lots of success and keeping my fingers crossed for you.

And remember...you are the guru!

Other books by Sibel Hodge

Fourteen Days Later

Fourteen Days Later was short listed for the Harry Bowling Prize 2008 and received a Highly Commended by the Yeovil Literary Prize 2009. It is a romantic comedy with a unique infusion of British and Turkish Cypriot culture. Written in a similar style to Marian Keyes, it is My Big Fat Greek Wedding meets Bridget Jones.

When accident-prone Helen Grey finds a thong stuffed into the pocket of her boyfriend's best work trousers, it's time for her to move on. His excuse that he needed to dust the photocopier and just thought that it was a rag sounds like a lame excuse.

Helen's life is propelled in an unexpected direction after her best friend, Ayshe, sets her a fourteen-day, life-changing challenge. Helen receives a task everyday which she must complete without question. The tasks are designed to build her confidence and boost her self-esteem but all they seem to do is push her closer to Ayshe's brother, Kalem.

How will Kalem and Helen get together when she's too foolish to realize that she loves him? How can he fall for her when he is too busy falling prey to her mishaps and too in love with his own perfect girlfriend? How will Kalem's Turkish Cypriot family react when they find out?

Is it really possible to change your life in fourteen days?

My Perfect Wedding

Helen Grey is finally getting everything she wants. She's about to have the perfect dream wedding and begin an exciting new life abroad on the sunny Mediterranean island of Cyprus. But living the dream isn't all it's cracked up to be.

After a mix-up at the airport, Helen finds herself drawn into the midst of an elaborate plot to steal an ancient statue and assassinate a local businessman. And as if that wasn't bad enough, her wedding dress is AWOL, the statue seems to be cursed, and Helen is wanted by the police.

With the big day rapidly approaching, a roller-coaster of mishaps, misunderstandings, and disasters threatens to turn the newlyweds into nearlyweds.

Can Helen prevent an assassination, save the statue, and have the perfect wedding? Or will the day to remember turn into one she'd rather forget?

The Fashion Police

The Fashion Police was a runner up in the Chapter One Promotions Novel Competition 2010 and nominated Best Novel with Romantic Elements 2010 by The Romance Reviews. It is a screwball comedy-mystery, combining murder and mayhem with romance and chick-lit. Written in a similar style to Janet Evanovich and Harlan Coben, it is Stephanie Plum meets Myron Bolitar.

Amber Fox has been making too many mistakes lately and something's got to give...

For starters, Amber accidentally shoots Chief Inspector Janice Skipper and gets thrown off the police force. The only one who knows the truth about the incident is Amber, but no one will believe her.

After accepting a job as an insurance investigator from her ex-fiancé, Brad Beckett, it turns out that Brad thinks they've still got unfinished business and the job description includes sexual favours that come with a price.

When fashion designer, Umberto Fandango, goes missing, Amber becomes embroiled in a complicated case. But Amber's arch-enemy, Chief Inspector Skipper, is also investigating his disappearance, and it's a race against time for Amber to solve the mystery before Skipper does and get her old job back. And just when Amber thinks things can't get any worse, she's being stalked by some crazy mobsters.

Who is Umberto Fandango? Is he dead? And can Amber stay one step ahead and stay alive?

Be Careful What You Wish For

For fans of Janet Evanovich, Kate Johnson, and Gemma Halliday...

Armed with cool sarcasm and uncontrollable hair, feisty insurance investigator Amber Fox is back in a new mystery combining murder and mayhem with romance and chicklit...

Three deaths.
A safety deposit box robbery.
The boxing heavyweight champion of the world.

Somehow, they're all related, and Amber has to solve a four year old crime to find out why.

As she stumbles across a trail of dead bodies and a web of lies spanning both sides of the social divide, it's starting to get personal. Someone thinks Amber's poking her nose in where it's not wanted, sparking off a game of fox and mouse – only this time, Amber's the mouse.

Amber's forced to take refuge in the home of her ex-fiancé, Brad Beckett, and now it's not just the case that's hotting up. So is the bedroom...

All Levi Carter wanted to be was the boxing heavyweight champion of the world, but at what cost?

All Carl Thomas wanted was to be rich, but would his greed be his downfall?

All Brad Beckett wants is to get Amber back, but there's a reason for the ex word.

Be careful what you wish for...you might just get it.

252

How to Dump Your Boyfriend in the Men's Room (and other short stories)

Welcome to my world…

I'm an author of chicklit romances and mysteries. In my spare time I'm Wonder Woman! My world is sometimes wacky, quirky, and very accident-prone.

This is a collection of five humorous short stories – what I like to call true fiction. Some are true, some are fiction, and some are a mixture of both. I guess you have to decide which is which!

I often get asked if I'm like any of my characters in my novels, and I have to groan and say, yes. When you read these stories you'll realize how, and a lot of them have inspired scenes in my novels, although names have been omitted or changed to protect me against lawsuits!

Are you ready to find out "how to dump your boyfriend in the men's toilets", why "yoga is bad for your house", what the "S-Word has to do with your lady garden", why you need to "follow that goat", and whether "kismet" does really exist?

CPSIA information can be obtained at www.ICGtesting.com
Printed in the USA
BVOW012302260312

286136BV00008B/14/P